Workbook to Accompany

Cardiopulmonary Anatomy and Physiology

Essentials for Respiratory Care

Fourth Edition

Terry Des Jardins, M.Ed., R.R.T.
Department of Respiratory Care
Parkland College
Champaign, Illinois

DELMAR
THOMSON LEARNING™

Australia Canada Mexico Singapore Spain United Kingdom United States

DELMAR
THOMSON LEARNING

Workbook to Accompany Cardiopulmonary Anatomy and Physiology, Essentials for Respiratory Care, Fourth Edition by Terry Des Jardins

Health Care Publishing Director:
William Brotmiller

Executive Editor:
Cathy L. Esperti

Acquisitions Editor:
Candice Janco

Developmental Editor:
Marjorie A. Bruce

Editorial Assistant:
Maria D'Angelico

Executive Marketing Manager:
Dawn F. Gerrain

Channel Manager:
Jennifer McAvey

Project Editor:
Mary Ellen Cox

Production Editor:
James Zayicek

Art/Design Coordinator:
Jay Purcell

Printed in the United States of America
2 3 4 5 GP 05 04 03 02

For more information, contact Delmar,
3 Columbia Circle, PO Box 15015,
Albany, New York 12212-5015;

Or you can visit our Internet site at
http://www.delmar.com

Library of Congress Cataloging-in-Publication Data

ISBN: 0-7668-2535-3

CONTENTS

INTRODUCTION

This workbook is designed to enhance the learner's understanding, retention, and clinical application of the material presented in the textbook. The questions in the workbook parallel (in a step-by-step fashion) the information presented in the textbook. The student is asked to do such things as label and color illustrations, fill in the blanks, define terms, match answers, calculate equations, and write short answers.

The completed study questions serve as an excellent study tool to help the student review and prepare for chapter quizzes and exams. This workbook also gives the reader an opportunity to evaluate the degree of mastery of the material presented in the text. Although answering 75 percent of the questions correctly is considered an acceptable mastery level, study and review should continue until greater than 90 percent accuracy has been achieved. The student may wish to copy and maintain unanswered questions of various sections of the workbook for reuse and periodic self-assessment.

Terry Des Jardins

16. Label and color the following structures of the oral cavity:

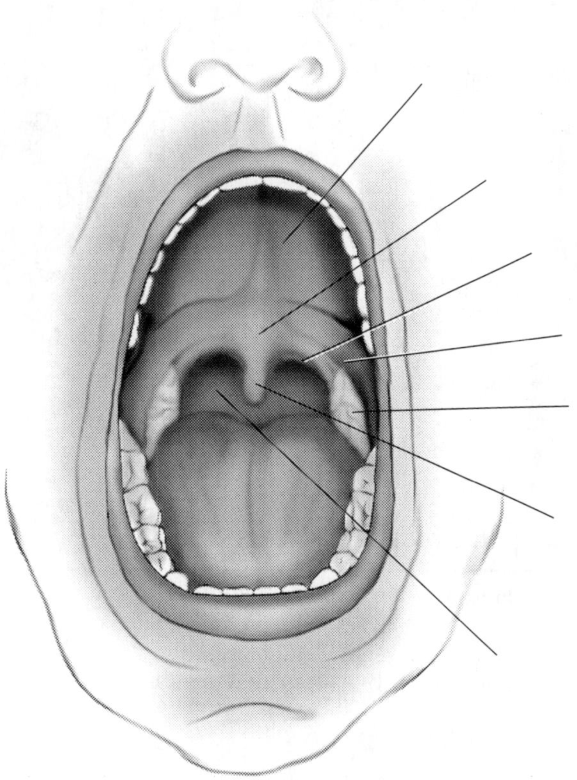

Figure 1–5 *Oral cavity.*

17. Functionally, the **larynx**:

a. ______________________________

____

b. ______________________________

____

c. ______________________________

____

18. Label and color the following cartilages of the larynx:

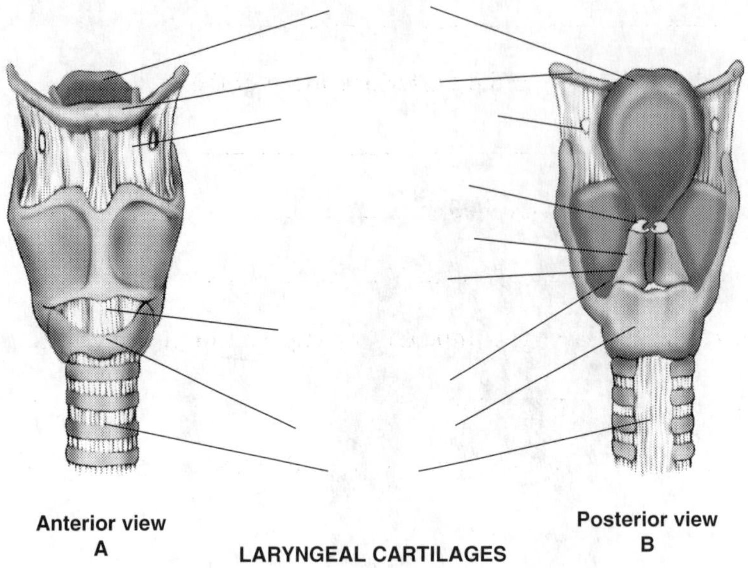

Figure 1–6 *Cartilages of the larynx.*

19. Label and color the structures observed in the superior view of the vocal folds:

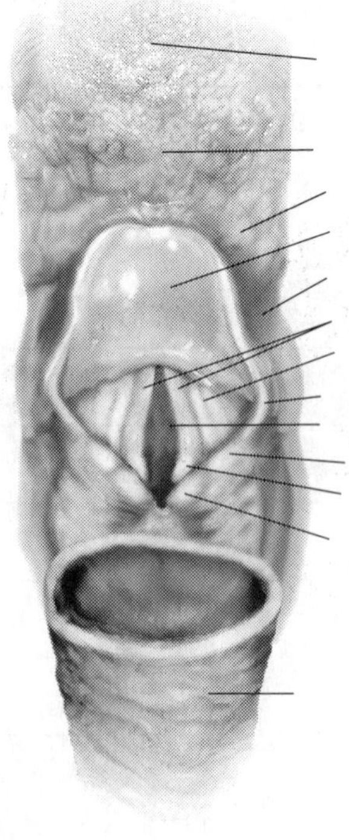

Figure 1–7 *A view of the base of the tongue, vallecula, epiglottis, and vocal cords.*

20. The elastic tissue that forms the medial border of each vocal fold is called the ________________

____.

21. Anteriorly, the vocal cords attach to the posterior surface of the ________________

____.

22. The space between the vocal cords is called the ________________________________

or the ____.

23. Above the vocal cords, the laryngeal mucosa is composed of ________________

________________ epithelium.

24. Below the vocal cords, the laryngeal mucosa is lined with ________________

________________ epithelium.

25. An expiratory effort against a closed glottis (e.g., during physical work such as lifting or pushing) is known as ____.

26. Label and color the following **extrinsic laryngeal** muscles:

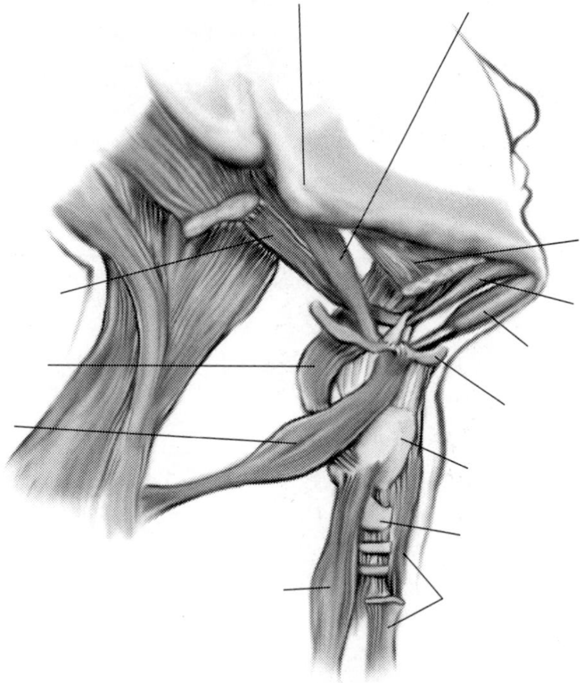

Figure 1–8 *Extrinsic laryngeal muscles.*

27. Label and color the following **intrinsic muscles** of the larynx:

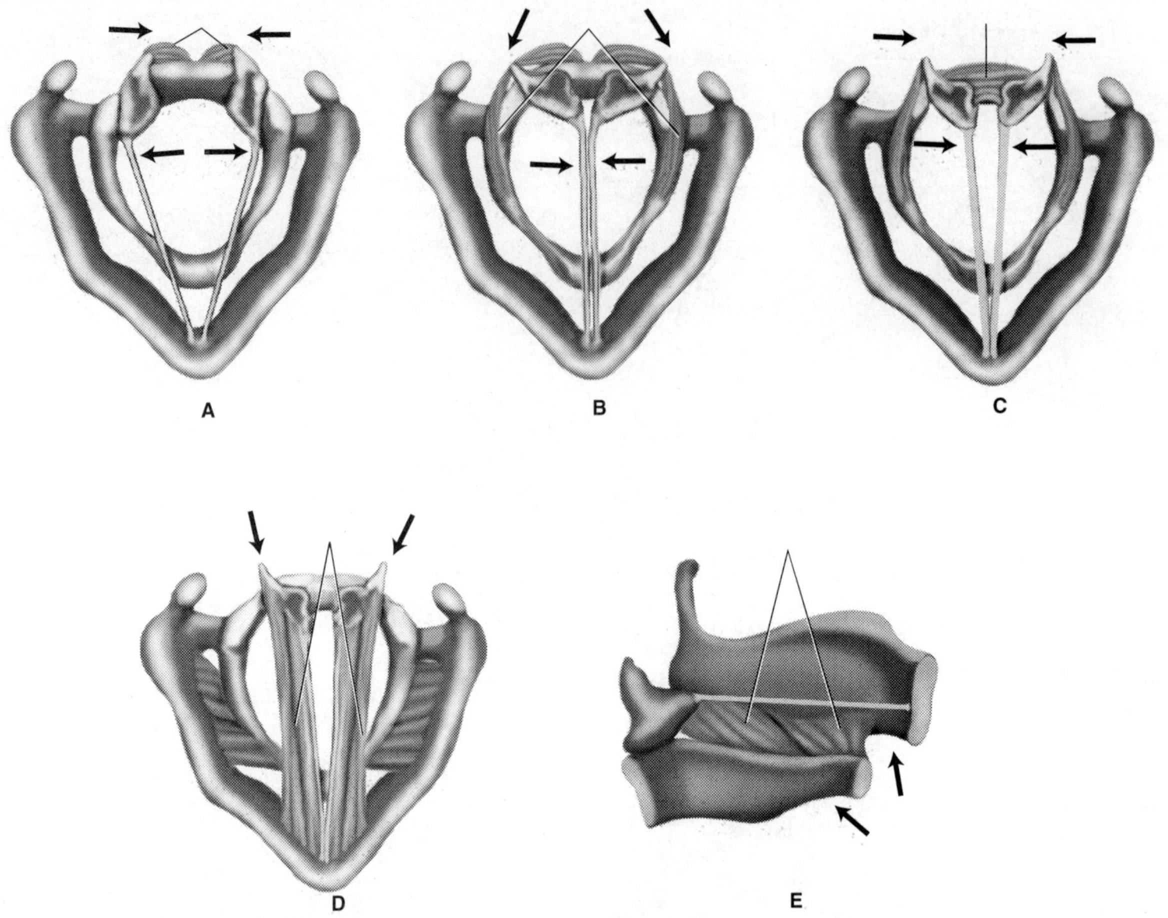

Figure 1–9 *Intrinsic laryngeal muscles.*

10. Label the following major structures around the lungs:

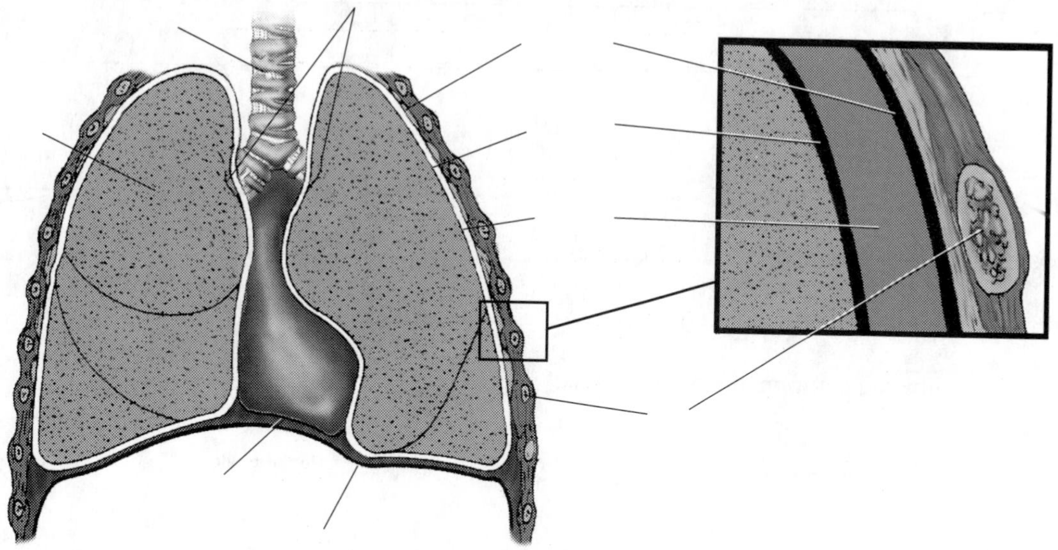

Figure 1–19 *Major structures around the lungs.*

THE MEDIASTINUM, PLEURAL MEMBRANES, AND THORAX

1. List the anatomic structures that are contained in, or pass through, the **mediastinum**:

___

___

___

2. The ______________________ pleura is firmly attached to the outer surface of each lung.

3. The ______________________ pleura lines the inside of the thoracic walls.

4. The potential space between the pleural membranes is called the ______________________

______________________.

List the three major structures that compose the sternum:

a. ______________________________

b. ______________________________

c. ______________________________

6. The first seven ribs are called the ______________________________.

7. Ribs eight, nine and ten are referred to as the ______________ ribs.

8. Ribs eleven and twelve are called the ______________ ribs.

9. Label the following components of the thorax:

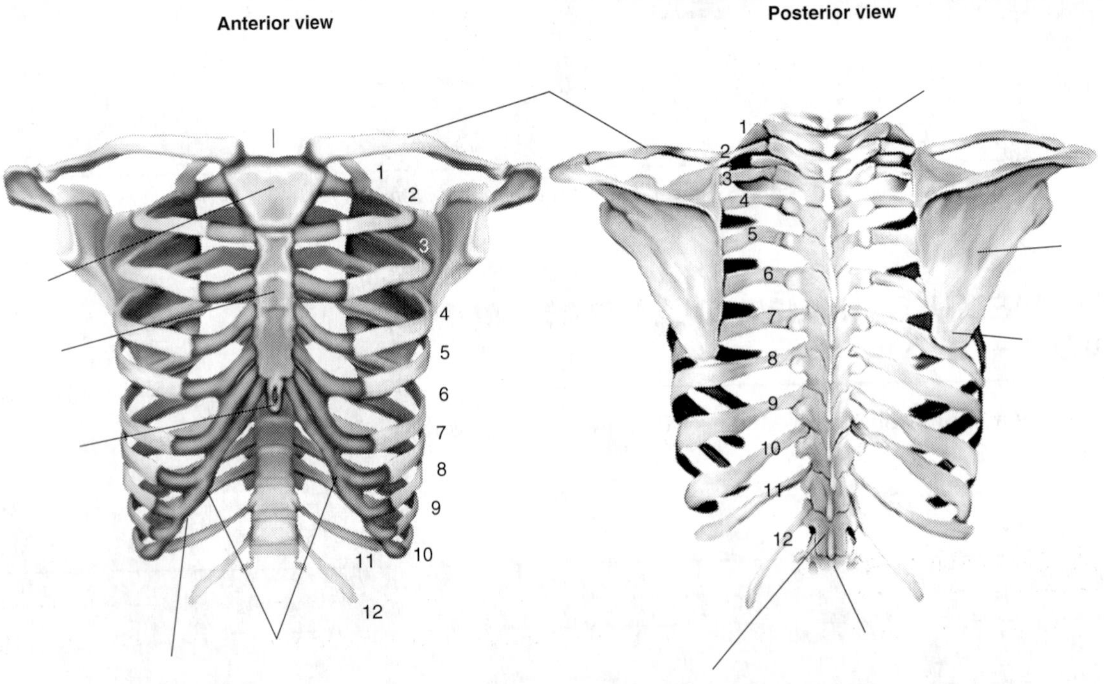

Figure 1–20 *The thorax.*

CHAPTER TWO

VENTILATION

PRESSURE DIFFERENCES ACROSS THE LUNGS

1. The pressure difference between two points in a tube or vessel is called the ______________________________________.

2. The barometric pressure difference between the mouth pressure and alveolar pressure is called the ______________________________________.

3. The difference between the alveolar pressure and the pleural pressure is called the ______________________________________.

4. The difference between the alveolar pressure and the body surface pressure is called the ______________________________________.

5. If the gas pressure at the beginning of a vessel is 12 mm Hg and the pressure at the other end of the same vessel is 7 mm Hg, what is the driving pressure?

Answer: ____________________

6. If the P_{alv} is 751 mm Hg and the P_m is 758 mm Hg, what is the P_{ta}?

Answer: ____________________

7. If the P_{pl} is 752 mm Hg and the P_{alv} is 748 mm Hg, what is the P_{tp}?

Answer: ____________________

8. If the P_{alv} is 751 mm Hg and the P_{bs} is 757 mm Hg, what is the P_{tt}?

Answer: ____________________

9. During inspiration, the thoracic volume increases and the intrapleural and intra-alveolar pressures ____________________.

10. During expiration, the intra-alveolar pressure is (_____ greater; _____ lower) than the barometric pressure.

11. During a normal expiration, the intrapleural pressure is always (_____ above; _____ below) the barometric pressure.

12. The normal intrapleural pressure change is about _____ to _____ cm H_2O pressure, or _____ to _____ mm Hg.

STATIC CHARACTERISTICS OF THE LUNGS

1. The term **static** refers to ____

____

____

2. The lungs have a natural tendency to (_____ collapse; _____ expand).

3. The chest wall has a natural tendency to (_____ collapse; _____ expand).

4. The two major static forces of the lungs are:

   a. ____

   b. ____

ELASTIC PROPERTIES OF THE LUNGS

1. **Lung compliance** is defined as the change in lung ____________________ per change in ________

____________________.

2. **Case A**

   a. If an individual generates an intrapleural pressure of -7 cm H_2O during inspiration, and the lungs accept a new volume of 385 ml of air, what is the compliance of the lungs?

   Answer: ____________________

b. If the same patient, four hours later, generates an intrapleural pressure of -5 cm H_2O during inspiration, and the lungs accept a new volume of 350 ml of air, what is the compliance of the lungs?

Answer: ____________________

c. The lung compliance of the above patient is (check one): increasing ____ decreasing ____

3. **Case B**

a. If a mechanical ventilator generates a $+9$ cm H_2O pressure during inspiration and the lungs accept a new volume of 450 ml of gas, what is the compliance of the lungs?

Answer: ____________________

b. If, on the same patient six hours later, the mechanical ventilator generates a $+15$ cm H_2O pressure and the lungs accept a new volume of 675 ml of gas, what is the compliance of the lungs?

Answer: ____________________

c. Compare the answers to the first two questions (a & b) above. The patient's lung compliance is (check one): increasing ____ decreasing ____

4. Under normal resting conditions, the average lung compliance during each breath is approximately

____________________.

5. According to the following volume-pressure curve, if an individual has a resting lung volume of 1500 ml, and generates a negative 25 cm H_2O pressure (in addition to the negative pressure required to maintain the resting lung volume), how many ml of gas will the lungs accommodate (in addition to the resting lung volume)?

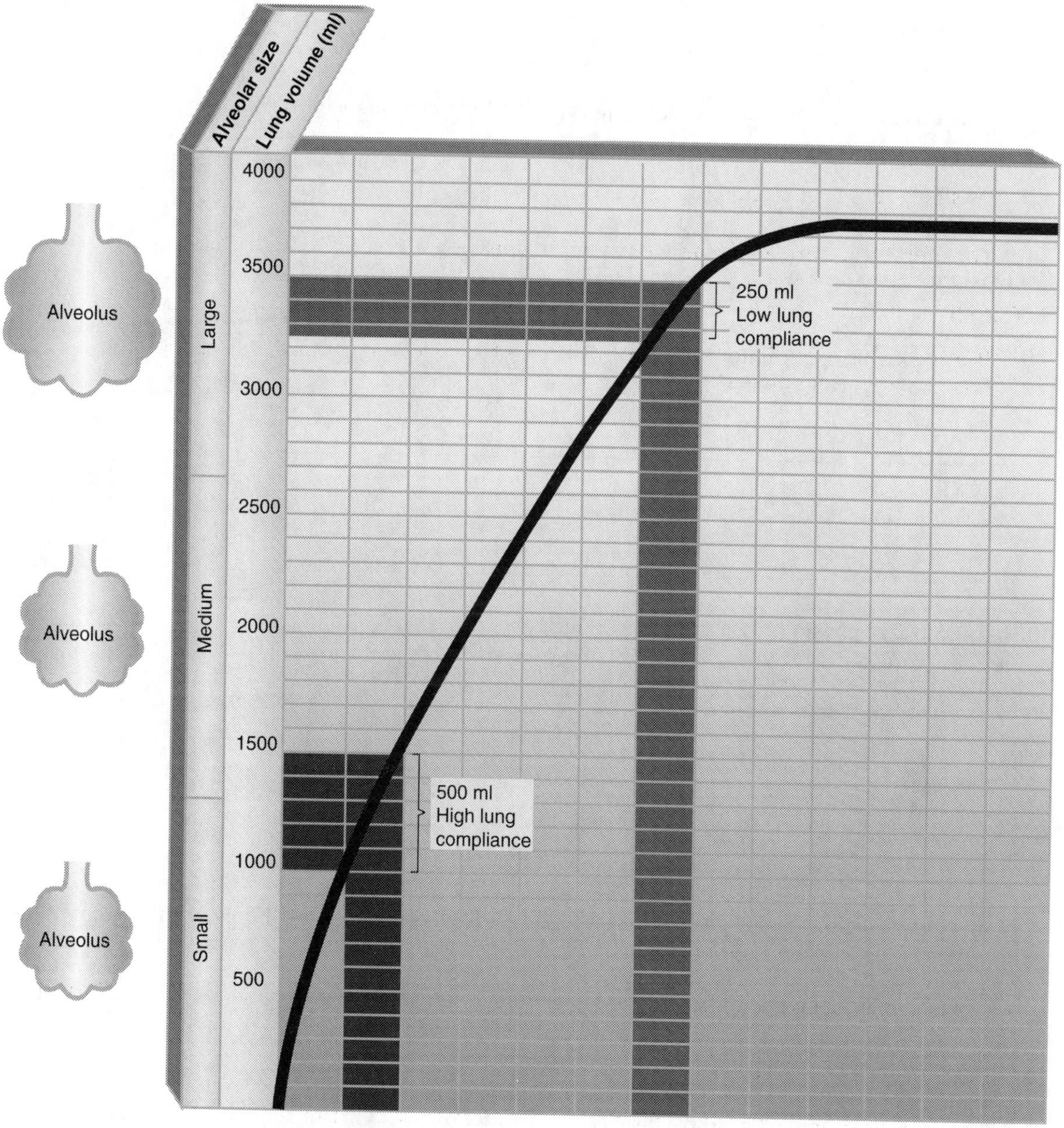

Figure 2–1 *Normal volume-pressure curve. The curve shows that lung compliance progressively decreases as the lungs expand in response to more volume. For example, note the greater volume change between 5 and 10 cm H_2O (small/ medium alveoli) than between 30 and 35 cm H_2O (large alveoli).*

Answer: ______________________

6. When lung compliance decreases, the volume-pressure curve moves to the ________________.

7. When the volume-pressure curve moves to the left, lung compliance is (circle one):

   a. increased
   b. decreased
   c. unchanged

8. As the alveoli approach their total filling capacity, lung compliance:

   a. increases
   b. decreases
   c. remains the same

9. **Elastance** is defined as ____

   ____

   ____

   ____

   ____

   ____

10. In pulmonary physiology, elastance is defined as ________________________
    and is expressed as:

    Elastance =

11. Lungs with high compliance have ________________ elastance, and lungs with low compliance

    have ________________ elastance.

12. **Hooke's law** states that ______________________________

____

____

____

____

____

13. When Hooke's law is applied to the elastic properties of the lungs, ______________________ is substituted for length and ______________________ is substituted for force.

14. The molecular, cohesive force at the liquid–gas interface is called ______________________.

15. The liquid film that lines the interior surface of the alveoli has the potential to exert a force of ______________________.

16. When Laplace's law is applied to a sphere with one liquid–gas interface, the equation is written as follows:

P =

17. The mathematical arrangement of Laplace's law shows that the distending pressure of a liquid bubble is

a. ______________________________

____

and

b. ______________________________

____

18. According to Laplace's law, as the surface tension of a liquid bubble increases, the distending pressure required to hold the bubble open ______________________; and as the radius of the bubble increases, the distending pressure ______________________.

19. When two different sized bubbles with the same surface tension are in direct communication the:

a. larger bubble will empty into the smaller bubble
b. smaller bubble will empty into the larger bubble
c. distending pressures in the two bubbles are equal; thus,there is no gas flow between the two bubbles.

20. During the formation of a new bubble, the principles of Laplace's law do not come into effect until the distending pressure of the liquid sphere goes beyond the ______________________.

21. As a liquid bubble increases in size, the surface tension:

a. increases
b. decreases
c. remains the same

22. **Pulmonary surfactant** is produced by the ______________________.

23. The surfactant molecule has both a hydrophobic end, which means it is ______________________, and a hydrophilic end, which means it is ______________________.

24. In the healthy lung, when the alveolus decreases in size, the amount of surfactant to alveolar surface area ______________________. This action causes the alveolar surface tension to ______________________.

25. It is estimated that the surface tension of the average alveolus varies from ______________________ in the small alveolus to about ______________________ in the fully distended alveolus.

26. List some general causes of surfactant deficiency:

a. ______________________
b. ______________________
c. ______________________
d. ______________________
e. ______________________

27. In the healthy lung, both the elastic force and the surface tension force are (______ low; ______ high) in the small alveolus.

DYNAMIC CHARACTERISTICS OF THE LUNGS

1. The term **dynamic** is defined as the ______________________________

____

2. In the lungs, dynamic refers to ______________________________

____

3. When **Poiseuille's law** is arranged for flow $\dot{V}$, it is written as follows:

$\dot{V}$ =

4. According to Poiseuille's law, and assuming all other variables remain the same:

   a. as the pressure increases, flow (______ increases; ______ decreases)

   b. as the length of a tube decreases, flow (______ increases; ______ decreases)

   c. as the radius of a tube increases, flow (______ increases; ______ decreases)

   d. as the viscosity decreases, flow (______ increases; ______ decreases)

5. Using Poiseuille's law equations and assuming all other variables remain the same, answer the following questions:

   a. If the radius of a tube that has gas flowing through it at 32 liters per minute (L/min) is reduced by 50 percent of its original size, what will be the new gas flow through the tube?

   Answer: ______________

b. If the radius of a tube that has gas flowing through it at 28 L/min is reduced by 16 percent, what will be the new gas flow through the tube?

Answer: ______________________

c. If the radius of a tube that has a driving pressure of 16 cm H_2O is reduced by 50 percent of its original size, what will be the new driving pressure required to maintain the same gas flow through the tube?

Answer: ______________________

d. If the radius of a tube that has a driving pressure of 10 cm H_2O is reduced by 16 percent of its original size, what will be the new driving pressure required to maintain the same gas flow through the tube?

Answer: ______________________

e. If the radius of a tube that has gas flowing through it at 50 L/min is increased by 50 percent of its original size, what will be the new gas flow through the tube?

Answer: ______________________

f. If the radius of a tube that has gas flowing through it at 100 L/min is increased by 16 percent of its original size, what will be the new gas flow through the tube?

Answer: ______________________

g. If the radius of a tube that has a driving pressure of 80 cm H_2O is increased by 50 percent of its original size, what will be the new driving pressure required to maintain the same gas flow through the tube?

Answer: ______________________

h. If the radius of a tube that has a driving pressure of 5 cm H_2O, is increased by 16 percent of its original size, what will be the new driving pressure required to maintain the same gas flow through the tube?

Answer: ______________________

6. Write the simple proportionalities of Poiseuille's law for flow ($\dot{V}$) and pressure (P):

$\dot{V}$=

P =

AIRWAY RESISTANCE AND DYNAMIC COMPLIANCE

1. Airway resistance (R_{aw}) is defined as the ______________________________

____

____

2. Write the equation for airway resistance (R_{aw}) and include the units of measurement:

$R_{aw} =$

3. If a patient produces a flow rate of 10 liters per second (L/sec) during inspiration by generating a transairway pressure (P_{ta}) of 30 cm H_2O, what is the patient's R_{aw}?

Answer: ______________

4. The normal R_{aw} in the tracheobronchial tree is about ____________ to ____________ cm H_2O/L/sec.

5. **Laminar** gas flow refers to ______________________________

____

6. **Turbulent** gas flow refers to ______________________________

____

7. **Time constant** is defined as the ______________________________

____

____

8. Lung regions that have an increased airway resistance, require:

   a. less time to inflate
   b. more time to inflate
   c. no change in time to inflate

9. Lung regions that have an increased compliance, require:

   a. less time to inflate
   b. more time to inflate
   c. no change in time to inflate

10. Which of the following causes lung regions to have a long time constant?

    I. Decreased airway resistance
    II. Increased lung compliance
    III. Increased airway resistance
    IV. Decreased lung compliance

    a. I only
    b. III only
    c. II and III only
    d. III and IV only
    e. II, III, and IV only

11. Lung regions that have a decreased airway resistance, require:

    a. less time to inflate
    b. more time to inflate
    c. no change in time to inflate

12. Lung regions that have a decreased compliance, require:

    a. less time to inflate
    b. more time to inflate
    c. no change in time to inflate

13. Which of the following causes lung regions to have a short time constant?

    I. Increased airway resistance
    II. Decreased lung compliance
    III. Decreased airway resistance
    IV. Increased lung compliance

    a. II only
    b. IV only
    c. III only
    d. I and IV only
    e. II and III only

14. **Dynamic compliance** is defined as the ______________________________

    ____

    ____

    ____

15. In the normal lung, the dynamic compliance is (_____ equal to; _____ greater than; _____ less than) static compliance at all breathing frequencies.

16. In the partially obstructed airways, the ratio of dynamic compliance to static compliance (_____ increases; _____ decreases; _____ remains the same) as the breathing frequency increases.

17. **Frequency dependent** refers to ______________________________

____

____

____

____

VENTILATORY PATTERNS

1. The **ventilatory pattern** consists of the following three components:

   a. ______________________________

   b. ______________________________

   c. ______________________________

2. The normal tidal volume is about _____ to _____ ml/kg; or _____ to _____ ml/lb.

3. The normal adult ventilatory rate is about _______ breaths per minute.

4. The normal I : E is about _____ : _____.

5. The gas that reaches the alveoli during inspiration is referred to as ______________________.

6. The gas that does not reach the alveoli during inspiration is referred to as ______________________

______________________.

7. **Anatomic dead space** is defined as ______________________________

____

____

____

8. If a patient weighs 130 pounds, about how many milliliters (ml) of inspired gas during each breath would be anatomic deadspace gas?

Answer: ____________________

9. **Alveolar ventilation** is equal to the ____________________ minus the ____________________ multiplied by the ____________________.

10. If an individual presents with this data:

- V_T = 575 ml
- V_D = 185 ml
- Breaths/minute = 16

What is the alveolar ventilation?

Answer: ____________________

11. **Alveolar deadspace** is defined as ____
____
____

12. **Physiologic deadspace** is defined as ____
____

13. In the upright position, the negative intrapleural pressure at the apex of the lung is normally (_____ less; _____ greater) than at the base.

14. In the upright position, the alveoli in the upper lung regions are (_____ smaller; _____ larger; _____ equal) in size compared to the alveoli in the lower lung regions.

15. In the upright lung, ventilation is much greater in the:

a. upper lung regions
b. middle lung regions
c. lower lung regions

16. When lung compliance decreases, the patient's ventilatory rate generally (____ increases; ____ decreases; ____ remains the same) and the tidal volume (____ increases; ____ decreases; ____ remains the same) .

17. When airway resistance increases, the patient's ventilatory rate generally (____ increases; ____ decreases; ____ remains the same) and the tidal volume (____ increases; ____ decreases; ____ remains the same) .

18. In response to a certain respiratory disorder, the patient may adopt a ventilatory pattern based on the expenditure of ______________________________ rather than the efficiency of ______________________________ .

19. **Apnea** is defined as the ______________________________

____

20. **Eupnea** is defined as ______________________________

____

21. **Biot's breathing** is defined as ______________________________

____

____

____

22. **Hyperpnea** is defined as ______________________________

____

____

23. **Hyperventilation** is defined as ______________________________

____

____

____

24. **Hypoventilation** is defined as ______________________________

____

____

____

25. **Tachypnea** is defined as ______________________________

____

26. **Cheyne-Stokes breathing** is defined as ______________________________

____

____

____

____

27. **Kussmaul breathing** is defined as ______________________________

____

____

28. **Orthopnea** is defined as ______________________________

____

____

____

29. **Dyspnea** is defined as ______________________________

____

____

CHAPTER THREE

THE DIFFUSION OF PULMONARY GASES

DIFFUSION AND GAS LAWS

1. **Diffusion** is defined as ______________________________

____

____

2. **Boyle's law** states that ______________________________

____

____

3. Boyle's law is written as follows:

4. If an airtight container, which has a volume of 400 ml and a pressure of 50 cm H_2O, has its volume reduced to 300 ml, what will be the new pressure in the container?

Answer: ____________________

5. If an airtight container, which has a volume of 55 ml and a pressure of 75 cm H_2O, has its volume increased to 110 ml, what will be the new pressure in the container?

Answer: ____________________

6. **Charles' law** states that ____________________

____

____

____

7. Charles' law is written as follows:

8. If the temperature of gas in an 8-liter balloon is increased from 290 Kelvin to 340 Kelvin, what will be the new volume in the balloon?

Answer: ______________________

9. If the temperature of an automobile tire, which has 4.5 liters of air in it, is increased from 32° Celsius to 42° Celsius, what will be the new volume of gas (air) in the tire?

Answer: ______________________

10. **Gay-Lussac's law** states that ____

____

____

____

11. Gay-Lussac's law is written as follows:

12. If the temperature of gas in a closed container, which has a pressure of 15 cm H_2O, is increased from 360 Kelvin to 375 Kelvin, what will be the new pressure in the container?

Answer: ______________________

13. If the temperature of the gas in a closed container, which has a pressure of 46 cm H_2O, is decreased from 40° Celsius to 30° Celsius, what will be the new pressure in the container?

Answer: ______________________

14. **Dalton's law** states that ____

____

____

____

15. The following gases and their respective pressures are enclosed in a container:

GAS	PARTIAL PRESSURE
Nitrogen	470 mm Hg
Oxygen	130 mm Hg
Carbon Dioxide	50 mm Hg

According to Dalton's law, what is the total pressure in the container?

Answer: ______________________

THE PARTIAL PRESSURES OF ATMOSPHERIC GASES

1. At sea level, identify the percentage of the atmosphere and the partial pressure of the following gases that compose the barometric pressure:

TABLE 3–1 Gases That Compose the Barometric Pressure

GAS	% OF ATMOSPHERE	PARTIAL PRESSURE (mm Hg)
Nitrogen (N_2)		
Oxygen (O_2)		
Argon (Ar)		
Carbon Dioxide (CO_2)		

2. As one ascends a mountain, the barometric pressure (_____ increases; _____ decreases; _____ remains the same) and the percent concentration of oxygen (_____ increases; _____ decreases; _____ remains the same).

3. Compare the partial pressure of gases in the dry air, alveoli, arterial blood, and venous blood:

TABLE 3–2 Partial Pressure (in mm Hg) of Gases in the Air, Alveoli, and Blood

GASES	DRY AIR	ALVEOLAR GAS	ARTERIAL BLOOD	VENOUS BLOOD
P_{O_2}				
P_{CO_2}				
P_{H_2O} (water vapor)				
P_{N_2} (and other gases in minute quantities)				
Total				

4. The reason the partial pressure of oxygen in the atmosphere is so much higher than the partial pressure of oxygen in the alveoli is because

____

____

____

____

5. At body temperature, the alveolar gas has an absolute humidity of ____________ and a water vapor pressure (P_{H_2O}) of ________________________.

6. If a patient is receiving an $F_{I_{O_2}}$ of 0.70 on a day when the barometric pressure is 748 mm Hg, and if the Pa_{CO_2} is 50 mm Hg, what is the patient's alveolar oxygen tension ($P_{A_{O_2}}$)?

Answer: ________________

THE DIFFUSION OF PULMONARY GASES

1. List the structures of the alveolar-capillary membrane that gas molecules must diffuse through:

a. ________________________________

b. ________________________________

c. ________________________________

d. ________________________________

e. ________________________________

f. ________________________________

g. ________________________________

h. ________________________________

i. ________________________________

2. The thickness of the alveolar-capillary membrane is between ______________ to ______________.

3. In the healthy resting person, the average $P\bar{v}_{O_2}$ is __________ mm Hg and the average $P\bar{v}_{CO_2}$ is __________ mm Hg.

4. Under normal circumstances, when venous blood enters the alveolar-capillary system, there is an oxygen pressure gradient of about __________ mm Hg, and a carbon dioxide pressure gradient of about __________ mm Hg.

5. The equilibrium of oxygen and carbon dioxide in the alveolar-capillary system is usually accomplished in about __________ seconds.

6. The total transit time for blood to move through the alveolar-capillary system is about __________ seconds, which is about __________ of the time available.

7. During exercise, the time available for gas diffusion (circle one):

   a. increases
   b. decreases
   c. remains the same

8. **Fick's law** is written as follows:

   $\dot{V}$ gas α

9. According to Fick's law, as the

   a. thickness decreases, gas diffusion (circle one):

      a. increases
      b. decreases
      c. remains the same

   b. pressure difference increases, gas diffusion:

      a. increases
      b. decreases
      c. remains the same

c. area decreases, gas diffusion:

a. increases
b. decreases
c. remains the same

10. **Henry's law** states that: ____________________

____

____

____

11. The amount of gas that can be dissolved by 1 ml of a given liquid at standard pressure and specified temperature is known as the ____________________.

12. **Graham's law** states that the rate of diffusion of a gas through a liquid is

a. ____________________

____

____

and

b. ____________________

____

PERFUSION- AND DIFFUSION-LIMITED GAS FLOW

1. **Perfusion limited** means that ____________________

____

____

____

2. **Diffusion limited** means that ____

____

____

____

3. Under normal circumstances, the diffusion of oxygen is:

   a. perfusion limited
   b. diffusion limited
   c. neither perfusion nor diffusion limited

CHAPTER FOUR

PULMONARY FUNCTION MEASUREMENTS

LUNG VOLUMES AND CAPACITIES

1. **Tidal volume** (V_T) is defined as ______________________________

____

____

2. **Inspiratory reserve volume** (IRV) is defined as ______________________________

____

____

3. **Expiratory reserve volume** (ERV) is defined as ______________________________

____

____

4. **Residual volume** (RV) is defined as ______________________________

____

____

5. **Vital capacity** (VC) is defined as ______________________________

____

____

6. **Inspiratory capacity** (IC) is defined as ______________________________

____

____

7. **Functional residual capacity** (FRC) is defined as ______________________________

____

____

8. **Total lung capacity** (TLC) is defined as ______________________________

____

____

9. **Residual volume/total lung capacity ratio** (RV/TLC × 100) is defined as ______________

____

____

10. Compare the approximate lung volumes and capacities in the average normal male and female between 20 and 30 years of age:

TABLE 4–1 Approximate Lung Volumes and Capacities in the Average Normal Subject Between 20 and 30 Years of Age

	MALE		FEMALE	
MEASUREMENT	ml	Approx. % of TLC	ml	Approx. % of TLC
Tidal Volume (V_T)				
Inspiratory Reserve Volume (IRV)				
Expiratory Reserve Volume (ERV)				
Residual Volume (RV)				
Vital Capacity (VC)				
Inspiratory Capacity (IC)				
Functional Residual Capacity (FRC)				
Total Lung Capacity (TLC)				
Residual Volume/Total Lung Capacity Ratio (RV/TLC × 100)				

11. In an obstructive lung disorder, the ______________, ______________, ______________, and ______________ are increased; and the ______________, ______________, ______________ and ______________ are decreased.

12. In a restrictive lung disorder, the ______________, ______________, ______________, ______________, ______________, and ______________, are all decreased.

13. Because the *residual volume* (RV) cannot be exhaled, the RV, and lung capacities that contain the RV, are measured indirectly by one of the following methods:

a. ______

b. ______

c. ______

PULMONARY MECHANICS

1. **Forced vital capacity** (FVC) is defined as ______

2. **Forced expiratory volume timed** (FEV_T) is defined as ______

3. The normal percentage of the total volume exhaled during the following time periods is:

a. $FEV_{0.5}$ ______ %

b. $FEV_{1.0}$ ______ %

c. $FEV_{2.0}$ ______ %

d. $FEV_{3.0}$ ______ %

4. In obstructive disease, the percentage of FVC that can be forcefully exhaled over a specific period of time (______ increases; ______ decreases; ______ remains the same) .

5. Forced expiratory $volume_{1\ Sec}$/Forced vital capacity ratio (FEV_1/FVC ratio) is the ______

6. Because the FEV_1/FVC ratio is expressed as a percentage, it is commonly referred to as a ______

7. Under normal conditions the patient's $FEV_{1\%}$ shoud be ______________ or greater.

8. Collectively, the **FEV, FEV_1**, and the **$FEV_{1\%}$** are the most commonly used pulmonary function measurements to

   a. ____

   b. ____

9. In **obstructive lung disorders**, both the FEV_1 and the $FEV_{1\%}$ are (______ decreased, ______ increased).

10. In **restrictive lung disorders**, the FEV_1 is down, but the $FEV_{1\%}$ is ______________.

11. **Forced expiratory flow$_{25\%-75\%}$** ($FEF_{25\%-75\%}$) is defined as ____

____

____

____

12. The $FEF_{25\%-75\%}$ reflects the status of the ______________ to ______________ -sized airways.

13. **Forced expiratory flow$_{200-1200}$** ($FEF_{200-1200}$) is defined as ____

____

____

____

14. The $FEF_{200-1200}$ is a good index of the (______ large; ______ small) airway function.

15. **Peak expiratory flow rate** (PEFR) is defined as ____

____

____

16. **Maximum voluntary ventilation** (MVV) is defined as ____

____

____

17. Label the following measurements graphically presented in the **flow-volume loop**:

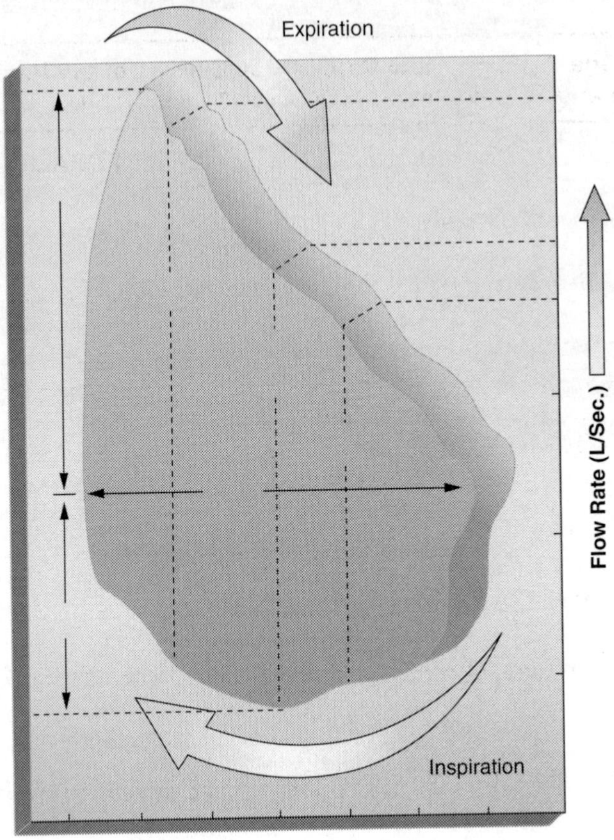

Figure 4–1 *Normal flow-volume loop. PEFR — peak expiration flow rate; PIFR — peak inspiratory flow rate; FVC — forced vital capacity;* $FEF_{25\%-75\%}$ *— forced expiratory* $flow_{25\%-75\%}$ *;* $FEF_{50\%}$ *— forced expiratory* $flow_{50\%}$ *(also called* $\dot{V}max_{50}$ *).*

18. Compare the following average dynamic flow rate measurements of the healthy male and female between 20 and 30 years of age:

TABLE 4–2 Average Dynamic Flow Rate Measurements of the Healthy Male and Female Between 20 and 30 Years of Age

MEASUREMENT	MALE	FEMALE
FEV_T		
$FEV_{0.5}$		
$FEV_{1.0}$		
$FEV_{2.0}$		
$FEV_{3.0}$		
$FEF_{200-1200}$		
$FEF_{25\%-75\%}$		
PEFR		
MVV		

EFFECTS OF DYNAMIC COMPRESSION ON EXPIRATORY FLOW RATES

1. During approximately the first 30 percent of a forced vital capacity (FVC) maneuver the maximum peak flow rate is ______________________________

____

2. The first portion if the FVC (First 30%) maneuver originates from the large airways and is referred to as ______________________________.

3. Approximately the last 70 percent of a forced vital capacity maneuver is effort independent. **Effort independent** means that:

____

____

____

4. The limitation of the flow rate that occurs during the last 70 percent of a forced vital capacity maneuver is caused by the ________________ of the walls of the airway.

5. As muscular effort and intrapleural pressure increase during a forced expiratory maneuver, the **equal pressure point** moves ________________.

6. Once dynamic compression occurs during a forced expiratory maneuver, increased muscular effort (____ increases; ____ decreases; ____ has no effect on) airway compression.

CHAPTER FIVE

THE ANATOMY AND PHYSIOLOGY OF THE CIRCULATORY SYSTEM

BLOOD

1. List the four major components of blood:

   a. ______________________________

   b. ______________________________

   c. ______________________________

   d. ______________________________

2. The ______________________ constitute the major portion of the blood cells.

3. In the healthy adult male, there are about ______________ million red blood cells in each cubic millimeter of blood.

4. In the healthy adult female, there are about ______________ million red blood cells in each cubic millimeter of blood.

5. The percentage of red blood cells in relation to the total blood volume is known as the ______________________.

6. Compare the normal hematocrit levels for the following:

   a. Adult male ________ %

   b. Adult female ________ %

   c. Newborn ______ to ______ %

7. Microscopically, the red blood cells appear as biconcave disks, averaging about ______________ in diameter and ______________ in thickness.

8. The life span of an RBC is about ______________ days.

9. The major function of the leukocytes is to ______________

____

____

____

____

10. The normal amount of leukocytes averages between ______________ to ______________ cells per cubic millimeter of blood.

11. Compare the normal differential count for the following:

TABLE 5–1 Normal Differential Count

POLYMORPHONUCLEAR GRANULOCYTES	MONONUCLEAR CELLS
Neutrophils	Lymphocytes
Eosinophils	Monocytes
Basophils	

12. The most numerous of the white blood cells are the ______________ ______________.

13. ______________ are commonly elevated in response to an allergic condition.

14. The ______________ play an important role in immunity.

15. ______________ are commonly elevated in response to a chronic infection.

16. Thrombocytes are also called ______________.

17. The normal platelet count in each cubic millimeter of blood ranges between ______________ and ______________.

18. The function of the platelets is to ______________

____

____

____

19. Plasma constitutes about ______________ percent of the total blood volume.

20. Approximately ______________ percent of the plasma consists of water.

21. List the three types of **proteins** found in the plasma:

a. ______________

b. ______________

c. ______________

22. List the **electrolyte cations** found in the plasma:

a. ______________

b. ______________

c. ______________

d. ______________

23. List the **electrolyte anions** found in the plasma:

a. ______________

b. ______________

c. ______________

d. ______________

24. List the four types of **food substances** found in the plasma:

a. ______

b. ______

c. ______

d. ______

25. List the four types of **waste products** found in the plasma:

a. ______

b. ______

c. ______

d. ______

THE HEART

1. Label and color the following anatomic structures of the heart:

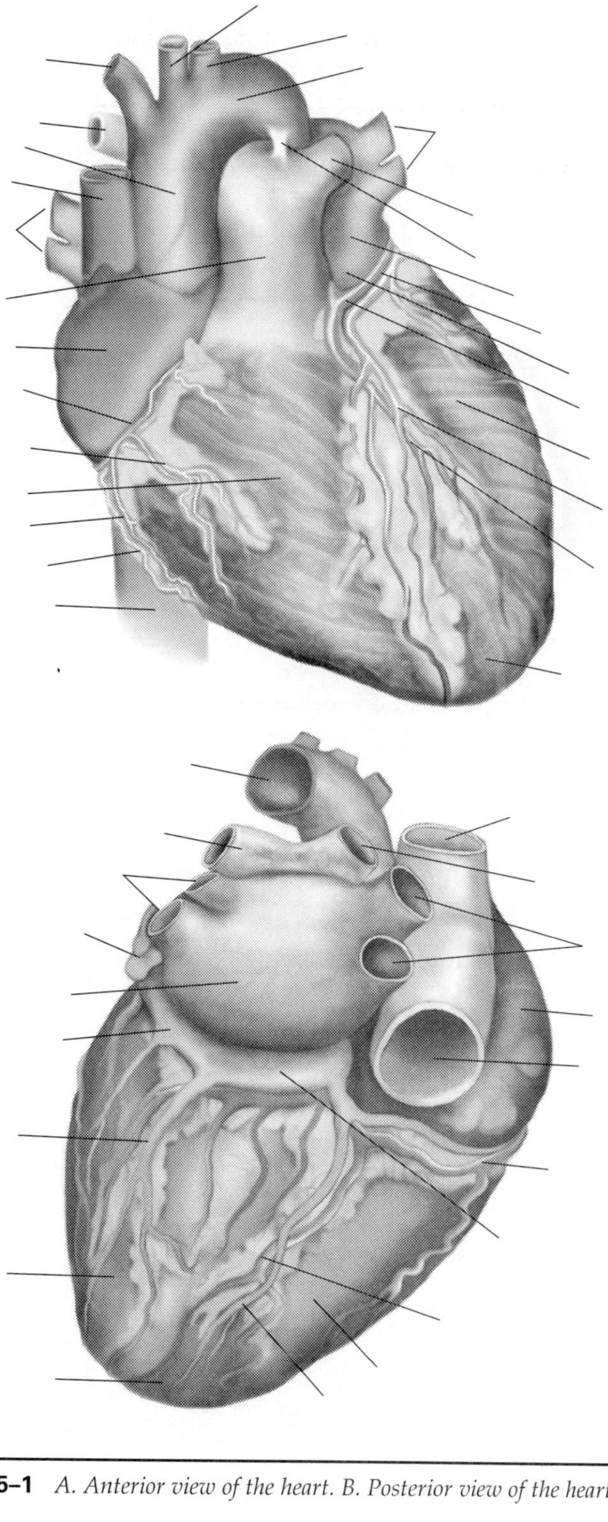

Figure 5–1 *A. Anterior view of the heart. B. Posterior view of the heart.*

2. The **heart** is a hollow, four-chambered, muscular organ that continually propels oxygen and nutrients, and consists of the upper right and left ______________ and the lower right and left ______________.

3. The atria are separated by a thin muscular wall called the ______________; the ventricles are separated by a thick muscular wall called the ______________.

4. The right atrium and ventricle act as one pump to propel ______________.

5. The left atrium and ventricle act as another pump to propel ______________.

6. The heart weighs between ________ and ________ grams.

7. When fingers are pressed between the fifth and sixth ribs just below the left nipple, the heartbeat can be felt where the apex is in contact with the internal portion of the chest. Clinically, this site is called the ______________.

The Pericardium

1. The heart is enclosed in a double-walled sac called the ______________.

2. The primary function of the **fibrous pericardium** is to:

   a. ______________

   b. ______________

   c. ______________

3. The inner wall, called the **serous pericardium**, is composed of two layers; the ______________, and the ______________.

THE WALL OF THE HEART

1. The **epicardium**, or visceral layer of the pericardium, is composed of ______________________________

____.

2. The **myocardium** consists of ______________________________

____.

3. The **endocardium** is located in the ______________________________

____.

BLOOD SUPPLY OF THE HEART

1. The blood supply that nourishes the heart originates directly from the aorta by means of two arteries—the ______________________________ and

____.

2. The *left coronary artery* divides into the ______________________________ and

____.

3. The *right coronary artery* supplies the right atrium and then divides into the ______________

______________________________ and ______________________________

____.

4. Venous blood from the anterior side of the heart empties into the ______________________________

____.

5. Venous blood from the posterior position of the heart is collected by the ______________________

____.

6. The great and middle cardiac veins merge and empty into a large venous cavity within the posterior wall of the right atrium, called the ______________________________.

7. A small amount of venous blood is collected by the ______________________, which empties directly into both the right and left atrium.

BLOOD FLOW THROUGH THE HEART

1. The right atrium receives venous blood from the ______________________ and ______________________.

2. A small amount of cardiac venous blood enters the right atrium by means of the ______________________.

3. A one-way valve called the ______________________ lies between the right atrium and the right ventricle.

4. The tricuspid leaflets are held in place by tendinous cords called ______________________.

5. The chordae tendineae are secured to the ventricular wall by the ______________________.

6. When the ventricles contract, the tricuspid valve closes and blood leaves the right ventricle through the ______________________ and enters the lungs by way of the right and left ______________________.

7. The ______________________ separates the right ventricle from the pulmonary trunk.

8. After blood passes through the lungs, it returns to the left atrium by way of the ______________________.

9. The ______________________ lies between the left atrium and the left ventricle.

10. The left ventricle pumps blood through the ascending ______________________.

THE PULMONARY AND SYSTEMIC VASCULAR SYSTEMS

1. The pulmonary circulation system begins with the ______________________ and ends in the ______________________.

2. The systemic circulation system begins with the ______________________ and ends in the ______________________.

3. The arteries are vessels that carry blood (_____ to; _____ away from) the heart.

4. The arteries subdivide into smaller vessels called ______________________.

5. The ______________ play a major role in the distribution and regulation of blood pressure.

6. Which vessels are referred to as the resistance vessels?

   Answer: ______________________.

7. In the capillaries of the pulmonary system, gas exchange is called ______________ respiration.

8. In the capillaries of the systemic system, gas exchange is called ______________ respiration.

9. Tiny vessels continuous with the capillaries are called ______________________.

10. Veins are also known as ______________________ vessels.

11. Approximately _____ percent of the body's total blood volume is contained within the venous system.

12. The pulmonary arterioles and most of the arterioles in the systemic circulation are controlled by ______________ impulses.

13. The ______________ center, located in the ______________, governs the number of ______________ impulses sent to the vascular systems.

14. Under normal circumstances, a continual stream of ______________ impulses are sent to blood vessels.

15. A moderate state of constant vascular constriction is called ______________________.

16. When the vasomotor center is activated to constrict a particular vascular region, it does so by (_____ increasing; _____ decreasing) the number of ______________ impulses sent to that vascular area.

17. When the vasomotor center causes vasodilation, it does so by (_____ increasing; _____ decreasing) the number of ________________ impulses sent to that vascular region.

18. List the major vascular beds in the systemic system that dilate in response to sympathetic impulses:

The arterioles of the:

a. ________________

b. ________________

c. ________________

19. **Baroreceptors**, which are specialized stretch receptors, are also called ________________ ________________.

20. The baroreceptors located in the carotid arteries send neural impulses to the medulla by means of the ________________ nerve.

21. The baroreceptors located in the arch of the aorta send neural impulses to the medulla by means of the ________________ nerve.

22. When the arterial blood pressure decreases, neural impulses to the medulla (_____ increase; _____ decrease), which, in turn, causes the medulla to (_____ increase; _____ decrease) its sympathetic activity.

23. When the baroreceptors signal the medulla to increase its sympathetic activity, the net result is:

a. ________________
____

b. ________________
____

c. ________________

____

24. In addition to the baroreceptors located in the carotid sinuses and aortic arch, other baroreceptors are found in the:

    a. ____

    b. ____

    c. ____

    d. ____

PRESSURES IN THE PULMONARY AND SYSTEMIC VASCULAR SYSTEMS

1. **Intravascular pressure** is defined as the ____

____

____

____

2. **Transmural pressure** is defined as the ____

____

____

____

3. A positive transmural pressure is when pressure inside the vessel is (_____ greater than; _____ less than; _____ the same as) the pressure outside the vessel.

4. A negative transmural pressure is when the pressure inside the vessel is (_____ greater than; _____ less than; _____ the same as) the pressure outside the vessel.

5. **Driving pressure** is defined as the ____

____

____

____

THE CARDIAC CYCLE AND ITS EFFECT ON BLOOD PRESSURE

1. The maximum pressure generated during ventricular contraction is the ____________________.
2. When the ventricles relax, the lowest pressure that remains in the arteries prior to the next ventricular contraction is the ______________________________.
3. Compared to the pulmonary circulation, the minimum pressure in the systemic system is about ______________ times greater.
4. Using the illustration below, identify the following mean intraluminal blood pressures at various points in the pulmonary and systemic circulation:
5. Normally, the stroke volume ranges between ______________ and ______________.
6. The total volume of blood discharged from the ventricles per minute is called ______________ ______________________.
7. If an individual has a stroke volume of 55 mL, and a heart rate of 80 beats per minute (beats/min), what is the cardiac output?

   Answer: ______________________________

8. Under normal conditions, when either the stroke volume or heart rate increases, the blood pressure:

   a. increases
   b. decreases
   c. remains the same

9. The normal adult total blood volume is about ____________ liters.

10. In regard to the total blood volume of the normal adults, about ______ percent is in the systemic circulation, ______ percent is in the heart, and ______ percent is in the pulmonary circulation.

11. Overall, about ______ percent of the total blood volume is in the veins, and about ______ percent is in the arteries.

THE DISTRIBUTION OF PULMONARY BLOOD FLOW

1. The fact that blood is **gravity dependent** means that it naturally moves ____________________

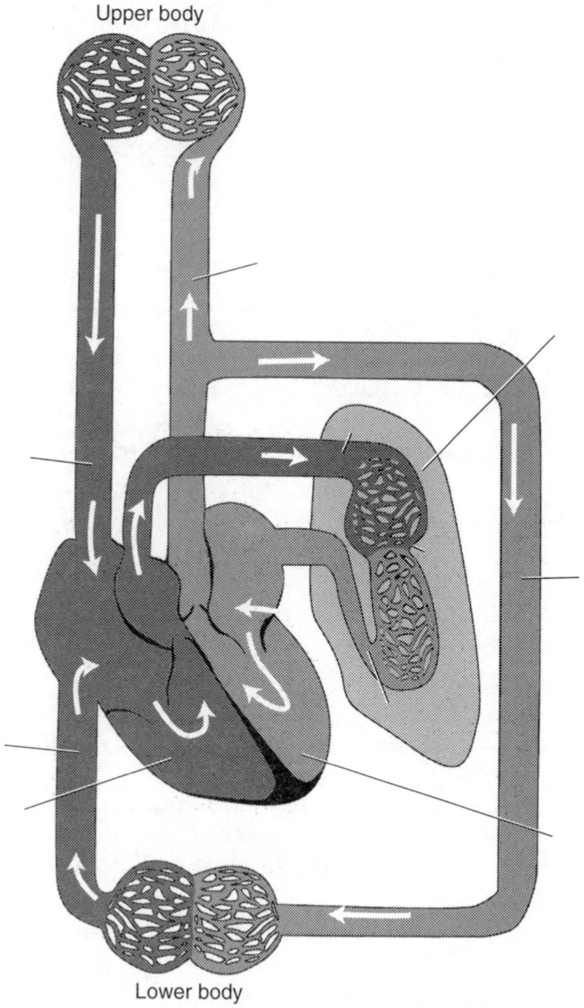

Figure 5–2 *Mean intraluminal blood pressure at various points in the pulmonary and systemic circulation.*

____

____

____

2. The intraluminal pressures in the vessels of the gravity-dependent areas of the lung are (_____ greater than; _____ less than; _____ the same as) the intraluminal pressures in the least gravity-dependent areas.

3. When an individual is in each of the following positions, which part of the lung is the gravity-dependent region?

BODY POSITION	GRAVITY-DEPENDENT LUNG REGION
a. Lying on the back	______________
b. Lying on the stomach	______________
c. Lying on the side	______________
d. Suspended upside down	______________

4. In **zone 1** of the upright lung, the alveolar pressure is sometimes (_____ greater than; _____ less than; _____ the same as) both the arterial and the venous intraluminal pressures.

5. List some conditions that can cause the alveolar pressure to be higher than the arterial and venous pressures:

   a. ____

   b. ____

   c. ____

6. When the alveoli are ventilated but not perfused, ______________________ is said to exist.

7. In **zone 2** of the upright lung, the arterial intraluminal pressure is (_____ greater than; _____ less than; _____ the same as) the alveolar pressure; and the alveolar pressure is (_____ greater than; _____ less than; _____ the same as) the venous pressure.

8. In **zone 3** of the upright lung, the arterial intraluminal pressure is (____ greater than; ____ less than; ____ the same as) the alveolar pressure; and the alveolar pressure is (____ greater than; ____ less than; ____ the same as) the venous pressure.

9. List the three mechanisms that determine stroke volume:

   a. ______________________________

   b. ______________________________

   c. ______________________________

10. **Ventricular preload** refers to ______________________________

    ____

    ____

11. Within limits, the more myocardial fiber is stretched during diastole, the (____ more; ____ less) strongly it will contract during systole.

12. **VEDP** stands for ______________________________

13. **VEDV** stands for ______________________________

14. As the VEDV increases the VEDP:

    a. increases
    b. decreases
    c. remains the same

15. The relationship between the VEDP and cardiac output is known as the ______________________________

    ____

16. **Ventricular afterload** is defined as ______________________________

    ____

    ____

17. Ventricular afterload is determined by:

    a. ______________________________

    ____

b. ______________________________

____

c. ______________________________

____

18. Clinically, what reflects the ventricular afterload the best?

Answer: ______________________________

19. **Blood pressure** (BP) equals:

BP = __________ × __________

20. **Myocardial contractility** can be pictured as ______________________________

____

____

____

21. In general, when the contractility of the heart decreases, the cardiac output:

a. increases
b. decreases
c. remains the same

22. List some clinical assessments that reflect myocardial contractility.

a. ______________________________

b. ______________________________

c. ______________________________

d. ______________________________

23. An increase in myocardial contractility is referred to as ______________________________

______________________________.

24. A decrease in myocardial contractility is referred to as ______________________________

______________________________.

25. Circulatory resistance is derived as follows:

Resistance =

26. In general, when the vascular resistance increases, the blood pressure:

    a. increases
    b. decreases
    c. remains the same

ACTIVE MECHANISMS AFFECTING VASCULAR RESISTANCE

1. Define **active mechanism**: ______________________________

    ____

    ____

    ____

2. In response to a decreased alveolar oxygen pressure, the pulmonary vascular system:

    a. constricts
    b. relaxes
    c. remains the same

3. In response to an increased P_{CO_2} level, the pulmonary vascular system:

    a. constricts
    b. relaxes
    c. remains the same

4. In response to a decreased pH, the pulmonary vascular system:

    a. constricts
    b. relaxes
    c. remains the same

5. In response to an increased H^+ concentration, the pulmonary vascular system:

    a. constricts
    b. relaxes
    c. remains the same

6. List some pharmacologic agents that constrict the pulmonary vessels:

   a. ______

   b. ______

   c. ______

   d. ______

   e. ______

7. List some pharmacologic agents that relax the pulmonary vessels:

   a. ______

   b. ______

   c. ______

   d. ______

8. List some pathologic conditions that increase pulmonary vascular resistance:

   a. ______

   b. ______

   c. ______

   d. ______

PASSIVE MECHANISMS AFFECTING VASCULAR RESISTANCE

1. Define **passive mechanism**: ______

   ______

   ______

   ______

2. In response to an increased pulmonary arterial pressure, the pulmonary vascular resistance:

   a. increases
   b. decreases
   c. remains the same

3. The answer to the above question occurs because of recruitment, which entails ______________________

   ____

   ____

   and because of distension, which entails ______________________________

   ____

   ____

4. In response to an increased left atrial pressure, the pulmonary vascular resistance:

   a. increases
   b. decreases
   c. remains the same

5. At high lung volumes, the pulmonary resistance in the alveolar vessels is (_____ high; _____ low).

6. At high lung volumes, the pulmonary resistance in the extra-alveolar vessels is: (_____ high; _____ low).

7. At low lung volumes, the pulmonary resistance in the alveolar vessels is (_____ high; _____ low).

8. At low lung volumes, the pulmonary resistance in the extra-alveolar vessels is: (_____ high; _____ low).

9. At high lung volumes, the pulmonary vascular resistance in the corner vessels is: (_____ high; _____ low).

10. At low lung volumes, the pulmonary vascular resistance in the corner vessels is (_____ high; _____ low).

11. In response to an increased blood volume, pulmonary vascular resistance:
    a. increases
    b. decreases
    c. remains the same

12. In response to an increased blood viscosity, the pulmonary vascular resistance:
    a. increases
    b. decreases
    c. remains the same

CHAPTER SIX

OXYGEN TRANSPORT

OXYGEN TRANSPORT

1. Compare the normal ranges for the following blood gas values:

Table 6–1 Normal Blood Gas Values Ranges

BLOOD GAS VALUE	ARTERIAL	VENOUS
pH		
P_{CO_2}		
HCO_3^-		
P_{O_2}		

2. The term **dissolved** means that when a gas like oxygen enters the plasma, it ____

____

____

3. Clinically, which portion of the oxygen transport system is measured to assess the patient's partial pressure of oxygen (P_{O_2})?

Answer: ______________________

4. Complete the following exercise:

   a. If an individual has an arterial oxygen partial pressure (Pa_{O_2}) of 50 mm Hg, about how many ml of oxygen are dissolved in every 100 ml of blood?

   Answer: ______________________ ml O_2/100 ml of blood

   b. In regard to the above answer, what is the vol% of dissolved oxygen?

   Answer: ______________________

5. Vol% (volume percent) is defined as ____

____

6. Each red blood cell (RBC) contains approximately __________ million hemoglobin molecules.

7. The normal adult hemoglobin is designated as Hb __________.

8. In the normal adult hemoglobin, how many heme group(s) are there?

   Answer: ______________________

9. Write the reversible reaction of O_2 with Hb:

10. When two oxygen molecules are bound to one Hb molecule, the Hb is said to be ________ percent saturated with oxygen; an Hb molecule with one oxygen molecule is ________ percent saturated.

11. Hemoglobin bound with oxygen is called ______________________________________.

12. Hemoglobin not bound with oxygen is called ____________________________________ or ______________________________________.

13. The amount of oxygen bound to hemoglobin is (______ indirectly; ______ directly) related to the partial pressure of oxygen.

14. The **globin portion** of each hemoglobin molecule consists of ____________________

____

____

____

15. **Fetal hemoglobin** (HbF) has ____________ chains and ____________ chains.

16. Hemoglobin changed from the ferrous state to the ferric state is known as ____________________

____.

17. Compare the normal hemoglobin values for the following:

a. Adult male: ____________ g% Hb

b. Adult female: ____________ g% Hb

c. Average infant: ____________ g% Hb

18. Hemoglobin constitutes about ________ percent of the RBC weight.

19. Each gram percent (g%) Hb is capable of carrying about ________ ml of oxygen.

20. At a normal arterial oxygen pressure (Pa_{O_2}) the hemoglobin saturation (Sa_{O_2}) is only 97 percent because of the following normal physiologic shunts:

a. ____

____

b. ____

____

c. ____

____

21. Complete the following total oxygen transport exercises:

Case A

A 23-year-old female with severe asthma presents with the following clinical data:

Hb: 13 g%
Pa_{O_2}: 55 mm Hg
Sa_{O_2}: 85%
Cardiac output: 6 L/min

a. How much dissolved O_2 is the patient transporting in every 100 ml of blood?

Answer: ______________ ml O_2/100 ml blood (vol%)

b. How much O_2 is bound to the hemoglobin in every 100 ml of blood?

Answer: ______________ ml O_2/100 ml blood (vol%)

c. What is the total O_2 content of the arterial blood (Ca_{O_2})?

Answer: Ca_{O_2} = ______________ (vol% O_2; or ml O_2/100 ml blood)

d. As the Ca_{O_2} is in reference to 1/10 of 1 liter of blood, how many ml of O_2 are available for tissue metabolism in one liter of blood?

Answer: ______________ ml O_2/liter

e. As this patient has a cardiac output of 6 L/min, how many ml of O_2 are available for tissue metabolism in 1 minute?

Answer: ______________ ml O_2/min

Case B

A 62-year-old male with severe emphysema presents with the following clinical data:

- Hb: 18 g%
- Pa_{O_2}: 50 mm Hg
- Sa_{O_2}: 80%
- Cardiac output: 3.5 L/min
- $P\bar{v}_{O_2}$: 25 mm Hg
- $S\bar{v}_{O_2}$: 50%
- PA_{O_2}: 150 mm Hg

a. How much dissolved O_2 is the patient transporting in every 100 ml of blood?

Answer: ____________________ ml O_2/100 ml blood (vol%)

b. How much O_2 is bound to the hemoglobin in every 100 ml of blood?

Answer: ____________________ ml O_2/100 ml blood (vol% O_2)

c. What is the total O_2 content of the arterial blood (Ca_{O_2})?

Answer: Ca_{O_2} = ____________________ (vol% O_2; or ml O_2/100 ml blood)

d. As the Ca_{O_2} is in reference to 1/10 of 1 liter of blood, how many ml of O_2 are available for tissue metabolism in 1 liter of blood?

Answer: ____________________ ml O_2/liter

e. As this patient has a cardiac output of 3.5 L/min, how many ml of O_2 are available for tissue metabolism in 1 minute?

Answer: ____________________ ml O_2/min

f. What is the patient's total oxygen content of mixed venous blood ($C\bar{v}_{O_2}$)?

Answer: $C\bar{v}_{O_2}$ = ______________________ (vol% O_2; or ml O_2/100 ml blood)

g. What is the patient's total oxygen content of capillary blood (Cc_{O_2})?

Answer: Cc_{O_2} = ______________________ (vol% O_2; or ml O_2/100 ml blood)

OXYGEN DISSOCIATION CURVE

1. The **oxygen dissociation curve** illustrates the ______________________ of hemoglobin that is chemically bound to oxygen at each oxygen ______________________.

2. Clinically, the **flat portion** of the oxygen dissociation curve is significant because it illustrates that

   a. ____

   ____

   b. ____

   ____

   c. ____

   ____

3. Clinically, the **steep portion** of the oxygen dissociation curve is significant because it illustrates that

   a. ____

   ____

   ____

   b. ____

   ____

4. Using the oxygen dissociation curve nomogram below, answer the next two questions (a and b).

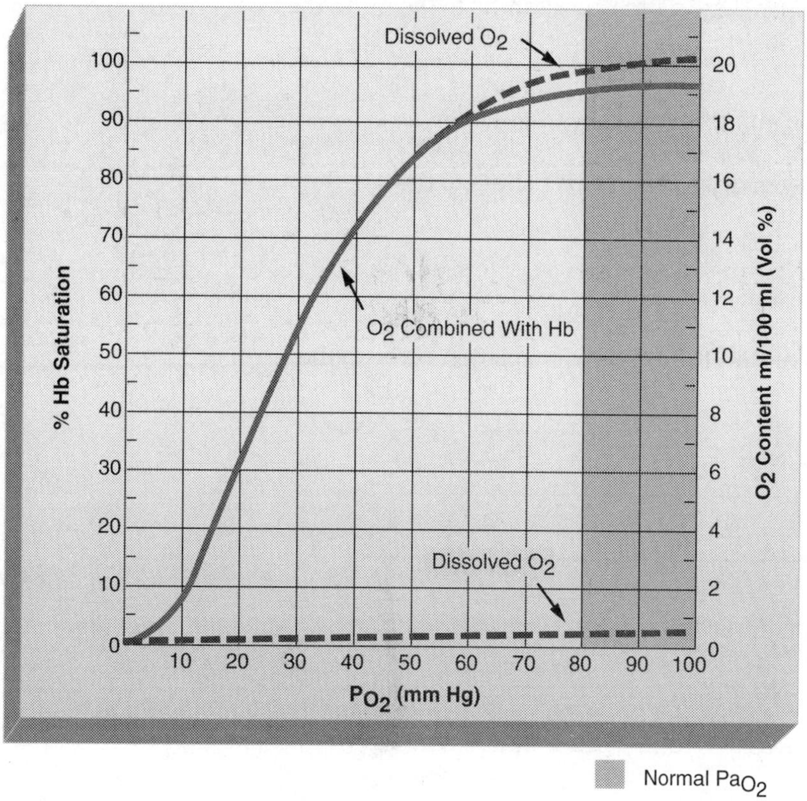

Figure 6–1 *Oxygen dissociation curve.*

a. If the P_{O_2} is 50 mm Hg, what is the percentage of hemoglobin that is bound to oxygen?

Answer: ___________________

b. What is the oxygen content level in vol%?

Answer: ___________________

5. The $\mathbf{P_{50}}$ represents ___________________

____

____

6. Normally, the P_{50} is about ______________ mm Hg.

7. When the oxygen dissociation curve shifts to the right, the P_{50}:

   a. increases
   b. decreases
   c. remains the same

8. When the oxygen dissociation curve shifts to the left, the P_{50}:

   a. increases
   b. decreases
   c. remains the same

9. List factors that shift the oxygen dissociation curve to the

   a. left: ______________________________

   ____

   ____

   ____

   ____

   ____

   b. right: ______________________________

   ____

   ____

   ____

10. Clinically, when the oxygen dissociation curve shifts to the *right*, the loading of oxygen in the lungs at any given P_{O_2}:

    a. increases
    b. decreases
    c. remains the same

11. Clinically, when the oxygen dissociation curve shifts to the *right*, the plasma P_{O_2} reduction necessary to unload oxygen at the tissue sites is:

    a. less than normal
    b. greater than normal
    c. the same as normal

12. Clinically, when the oxygen dissociation curve shifts to the *left*, the loading of oxygen in the lungs at any given P_{O_2}:

    a. increases
    b. decreases
    c. remains the same

13. Clinically, when the oxygen dissociation curve shifts to the *left*, the plasma P_{O_2} reduction necessary to unload oxygen at the tissue sites is:

    a. less than normal
    b. greater than normal
    c. the same as normal

OXYGEN TRANSPORT STUDIES

1. List the most common oxygen transport studies performed in the clinical setting:

    a. ______________________________
    b. ______________________________
    c. ______________________________
    d. ______________________________
    e. ______________________________
    f. ______________________________

2. **Total oxygen delivery** to the peripheral tissues is dependent on the:

    a. ______________________________
    b. ______________________________
    c. ______________________________

3. Complete the following formula:

$$\dot{D}_{O_2} =$$

4. If a patient has a cardiac output of 3.5 L/min and a Ca_{O_2} of 12 vol%, what is the total amount of oxygen delivered to the patient's peripheral cells?

Answer: ______________________

5. List three conditions that reduce an individual's total oxygen delivery:

a. ______________________

b. ______________________

c. ______________________

6. The **arterial-venous content difference** [$C(a - v)_{O_2}$] is defined as the difference ______________________

____

____

7. Complete the following formula:

$C(a - \bar{v})_{O_2} =$

8. If a patient has a Ca_{O_2} of 13 vol% and a $C\bar{v}_{O_2}$ of 9 vol%, what is the patient's $C(a - \bar{v})_{O_2}$?

Answer: ______________________

9. List some clinical factors that *increase* the $C(a - \bar{v})_{O_2}$:

a. ______________________________

b. ______________________________

1. ______________________________

2. ______________________________

3. ______________________________

4. ______________________________

10. List some clinical factors that *decrease* the $C(a - \bar{v})_{O_2}$:

a. ______________________________

b. ______________________________

c. ______________________________

d. ______________________________

e. ______________________________

11. The amount of oxygen extracted by the peripheral tissues during the period of one minute is called ______________________ or ______________________.

12. Complete the following formula:

$\dot{V}_{O_2} =$

13. If a patient has a cardiac output of 7.5 L/min and a $C(a - \bar{v})_{O_2}$ of 8 vol%, what is the patient's $\dot{V}_{O_2}$?

Answer: ______________________

14. List some clinical factors that *increase* the $\dot{V}_{O_2}$:

a. ______________________________

b. ______________________________

c. ______________________________

d. ______________________________

15. List some clinical factors that *decrease* the $\dot{V}_{O_2}$:

a. ______________________________

b. ______________________________

c. ______________________________

d. ______________________________

16. An individual's oxygen consumption index is derived by dividing the $\dot{V}_{O_2}$ by the ______________________________

____

17. The average oxygen consumption index ranges between ____________ and ____________ ml O_2/m^2.

18. The oxygen extraction ratio (O_2ER) is defined as the amount of oxygen

____

____

____

____

19. The O_2ER is also known as the

a. ______________________________

b. ______________________________

20. Complete the following formula:

$O_2ER =$

21. The normal O_2ER is ______________ percent.

22. a. If a patient has a Ca_{O_2} of 14 vol%, and a $C\bar{v}_{O_2}$ of 7 vol%, what is the patient's O_2ER?

Answer: ______________ percent

b. If the above patient has a total oxygen delivery of 850 ml/minute, then this would mean that during a course of 1 minute, ______________ ml of oxygen are metabolized by the tissues and ______________ ml of oxygen are returned to the lungs.

23. List some clinical factors that *increase* the O_2ER:

a. ______________

b. ______________

1. ______________

2. ______________

3. ______________

4. ______________

c. ______________

d. ______________

24. List some clinical factors that *decrease* the O_2ER:

a. ______________

b. ______________

c. ______________

d. ______________

e. ______________

f. ______________

25. The normal $S\bar{v}_{O_2}$ is ________ percent.

26. Clinically, an $S\bar{v}_{O_2}$ of about ________ percent is acceptable.

27. List some clinical factors that *decrease* the $S\bar{v}_{O_2}$:

a. ________________

b. ________________

1. ________________

2. ________________

3. ________________

4. ________________

28. A reduction in the $S\bar{v}_{O_2}$ indicates that the $C(a - \bar{v})_{O_2}$, $\dot{V}_{O_2}$, and O_2ER are:

a. increasing
b. decreasing
c. remaining the same

29. List some clinical factors that *increase* the $S\bar{v}_{O_2}$:

a. ________________

b. ________________

c. ________________

d. ________________

e. ________________

30. An increase in the $S\bar{v}_{O_2}$ indicates that the $C(a - \bar{v})_{O_2}$, $\dot{V}_{O_2}$, and O_2ER are:

a. increasing
b. decreasing
c. remaining the same

31. Indicate with the following code system how the clinical factors listed will likely alter a patient's total oxygen delivery, $\dot{V}_{O_2}$, $C(a-\bar{v})_{O_2}$, O_2ER, and $S\bar{v}_{O_2}$.

Code system: same = unchanged status; ↑ = increase; = ↓ decrease

Table 6–2 Clinical Factors Affecting Various Oxygen Transport Study Values

	OXYGEN TRANSPORT STUDIES				
CLINICAL FACTORS	D_{O_2} (1000 ml O_2/min)	$\dot{V}_{O_2}$ (250 ml O_2/min)	$C(a-\bar{v})_{O_2}$ (5 vol%)	O_2ER (25%)	$S\bar{v}_{O_2}$ (75%)
↑O_2 Consumption					
↓O_2 Consumption					
↓Cardiac Output					
↑Cardiac Output					
↓Pa_{O_2}					
↑Pa_{O_2}					
↓Hb					
↑Hb					
Peripheral Shunting					

MECHANISMS OF PULMONARY SHUNTING

1. **Pulmonary shunting** is defined as ______________________________

2. List the two major categories of conditions that cause a **true shunt mechanism**:

   a. ______________________________

   b. ______________________________

3. An **anatomic shunt** exists when ______________________________

4. The normal anatomic shunt is about __________ to __________ percent.

5. List three common causes of **anatomic shunting**:

   a. ______________________________

   b. ______________________________

   c. ______________________________

6. List three common causes of **capillary shunting**:

   a. ____

   b. ____

   c. ____

7. The sum of the anatomic and capillary shunts is referred to as ____________________ or ____________________.

8. What does **refractory** to oxygen therapy mean? ____________________

9. A **shunt-like effect** is said to exist when ____________________

10. List some common causes of the shunt-like effect mechanism:

    a. ____

    b. ____

    c. ____

11. What is **venous admixture**? ____________________

12. Complete the following shunt equation:

$$\frac{\dot{Q}_S}{\dot{Q}_T} =$$

13. A 42-year-old female is on a volume-cycled mechanical ventilator on a day when the barometric pressure is 740 mm Hg. The patient is receiving an $F_{I_{O_2}}$ of 0.45. The following clinical data are obtained:

Hb: 10 g%

Pa_{O_2}: 65 mm Hg (Sa_{O_2} = 91%)

Pa_{CO_2}: 35 mm Hg

$P\bar{v}_{O_2}$: 30 mm Hg ($S\bar{v}_{O_2}$ = 60%)

Using the information above, calculate the patient's $P_{A_{O_2}}$, Cc_{O_2}, Ca_{O_2}, and $C\bar{v}_{O_2}$.

a. $P_{A_{O_2}}$ =

Answer: ______________________

b. Cc_{O_2} =

Answer: ______________________

c. Ca_{O_2} =

Answer: ______________________

d. $C\bar{v}_{O_2} =$

Answer: ____________________

e. Using the clinical data above, calculate the patient's pulmonary shunt:

$$\frac{\dot{Q}s}{\dot{Q}T} =$$

Answer: ____________________

14. What is the clinical significance of the following calculated shunts:

a. below 10 percent: ____________________

____

b. 10–20 percent: ____________________

____

c. 20–30 percent: ____________________

____

d. greater than 30 percent: ____________________

____

15. List three clinical factors that cause the calculation of pulmonary shunting to be unreliable:

a. ____________________

b. ____________________

c. ____________________

TISSUE HYPOXIA

1. **Hypoxic hypoxia** is defined as ______________________________

____

____

2. List some conditions that can cause hypoxic hypoxia:

   a. ______________________________

   b. ______________________________

   c. ______________________________

3. **Anemic hypoxia** is defined as ______________________________

____

____

____

4. List two conditions that cause anemic hypoxia:

   a. ______________________________

   ____

   b. ______________________________

   ____

5. **Circulatory hypoxia** is defined as ______________________________

____

____

____

____

6. List two major forms of circulatory hypoxia:

   a. ____

   b. ____

7. **Histotoxic hypoxia** is defined as ____

8. Define **cyanosis**: ____

9. Define **polycythemia**: ____

CHAPTER SEVEN

CARBON DIOXIDE TRANSPORT AND ACID-BASE BALANCE

CARBON DIOXIDE TRANSPORT

1. List the three ways that carbon dioxide is transported from the tissue cells to the lungs in the **plasma**:

   a. ______________________________

   b. ______________________________

   c. ______________________________

2. List the three ways that carbon dioxide is transported from the tissue cells to the lungs in the **red blood cells**:

   a. ______________________________

   b. ______________________________

   c. ______________________________

3. In what form is most of the carbon dioxide carried to the lungs?

   Answer: ______________________________

4. The answer to the above question accounts for about ______ percent of the total amount of carbon dioxide transported to the lungs.

5. Using the following illustration, write the various chemical reaction(s) carbon dioxide goes through at the tissue sites to be transported to the lungs.

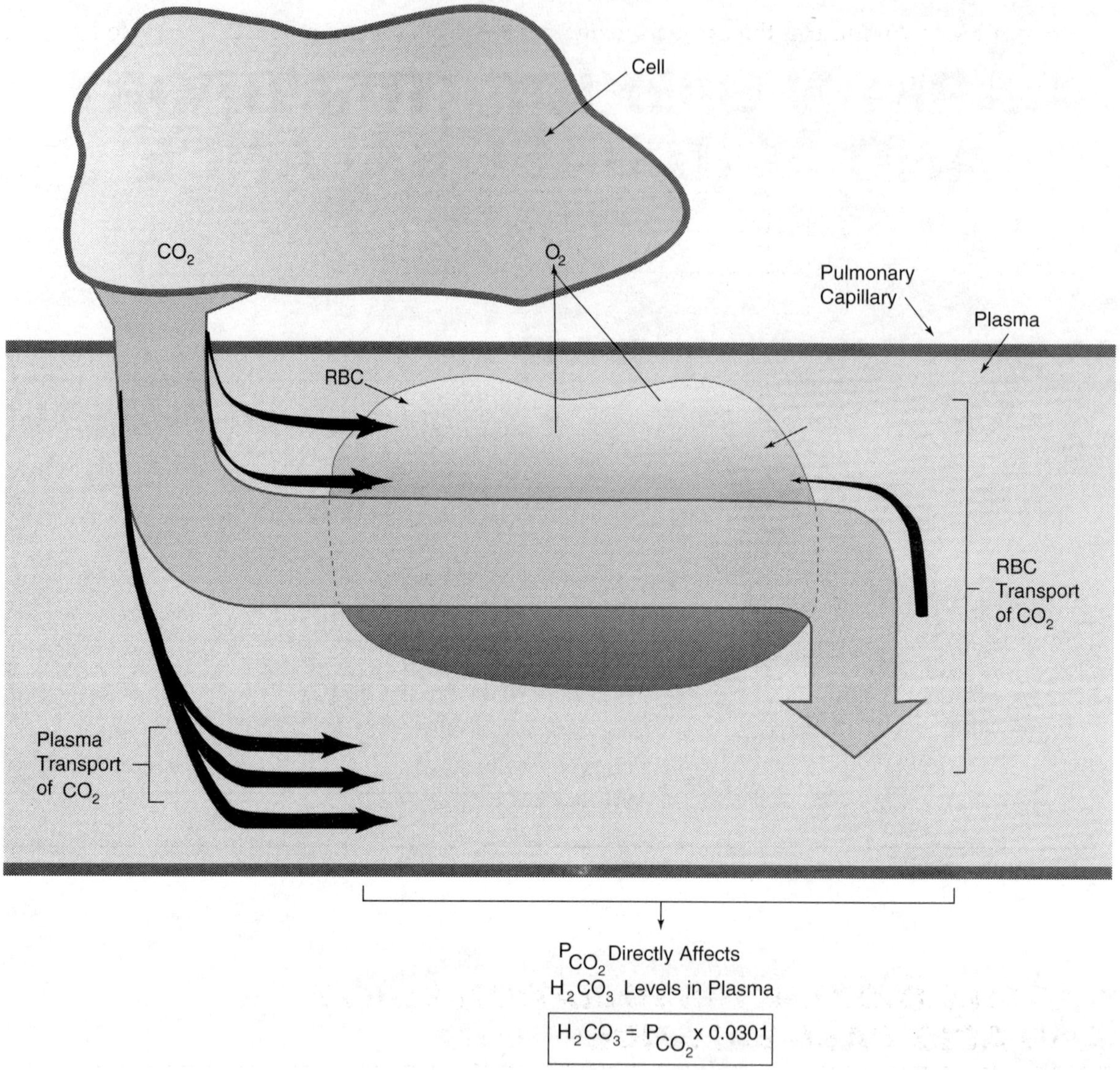

Figure 7–1 *How CO_2 is converted to HCO_3^- at the tissue sites. Most of the CO_2 that is produced at the tissue cells is carried to the lungs in the form of HCO_3^-.*

6. Unlike the S-shaped oxygen dissociation curve, the carbon dioxide curve is much more ________

____.

CARBON DIOXIDE ELIMINATION AT THE LUNGS

1. Using the following carbon dioxide dissociation curve nomogram, if the P_{CO_2} increases from 25 mm Hg to 40 mm Hg, the carbon dioxide content increases from ______ vol% to ______ vol%.

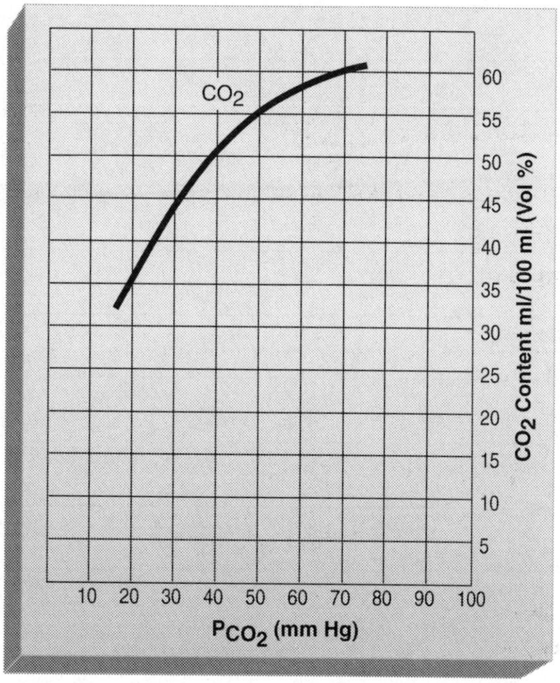

Figure 7–2 *Carbon dioxide dissociation curve.*

CARBON DIOXIDE DISSOCIATION CURVE AND ACID-BASE BALANCE

1. The fact that deoxygenated blood enhances the loading of carbon dioxide is called the ______________________________.

2. **Electrolytes** are ____

3. A **buffer** is a ______________________________

____

____

____

4. A **strong acid** is an acid that ______________________________

____

____

5. A **weak acid** is an acid that ______________________________

____

____

6. A **strong base** is a base that ______________________________

____

____

7. A **weak base** is a base that ______________________________

____

____

8. A **dissociation constant** refers to ______________________________

____

____

____

9. In the equation below, circle the portion of the acid or base system that is in the *dissociated state*:

$$HA \rightleftarrows [H^+] + [A^-]$$

10. A pH of 7 is ______________________.

11. A pH *less* than 7 is______________________.

12. A pH *greater* than 7 is ______________________.

13. In chemistry, the pH is defined as ____

____

____

14. The above definition of pH is written as:

pH =

15. A pH of 7 is equal to ______________ mol/L.

16. An *acid* is a substance that (_____ accepts; _____ donates) $[H^+]$.

17. An *acid* is a substance that (_____ increases; _____ decreases) the numerical value of the pH.

18. A *base* is a substance that (_____ accepts; _____ donates) $[H^+]$.

19. A *base* is a substance that (_____ increases; _____ decreases) the numerical value of the pH.

20. List the three mechanisms that maintain the narrow pH range:

a. ____

____

b. ____

____

c. ____

____

21. The most important buffer system in respiratory physiology is the ______________________

______________________combination.

22. The **Henderson-Hasselbalch equation** uses the components of the H_2CO_3/HCO_3^- system in the following way:

pH =

23. **pK** is derived from ____

____

____

24. Normally, the pK is ____.

25. The normal HCO_3^- to H_2CO_3 ratio is __________ to __________.

26. An HCO_3^- to H_2CO_3 ratio of 17 : 1 means the pH is:

   a. normal
   b. less than normal
   c. greater than normal

27. An HCO_3^- to H_2CO_3 ratio of 26 : 1 means the pH is:

   a. normal
   b. less than normal
   c. greater than normal

THE ROLE OF THE $P_{CO_2}/HCO_3^-/pH$ RELATIONSHIP IN ACID-BASE BALANCE

1. During acute ventilatory failure (hypoventilation), the blood (check one):

   a. P_{CO_2} (______ increases; ______ decreases; ______ remains the same)

   b. H_2CO_3 (______ increases; ______ decreases; ______ remains the same)

   c. HCO_3^- (______ increases; ______ decreases; ______ remains the same)

   d. HCO_3^- to H_2CO_3 ratio (______ increases; ______ decreases; ______ remains the same)

   e. pH (______ increases; ______ decreases; ______ remains the same)

2. In chronic ventilatory failure, the kidneys work to correct the pH status by:

   a. excreting HCO_3^-
   b. retaining H_2CO_3
   c. excreting H_2CO_3
   d. retaining HCO_3^-

3. In chronic ventilatory failure, partial or complete renal compensation can be verified when the HCO_3^- and pH readings on the $P_{CO_2}/HCO_3^-/pH$ nomogram are:

   a. greater than expected for a particular Pa_{CO_2}
   b. less than expected for a particular Pa_{CO_2}

4. During **acute alveolar hyperventilation** the blood (check one):

   a. P_{CO_2} (_____ increases; _____ decreases; _____ remains the same)

   b. H_2CO_3 (_____ increases; _____ decreases; _____ remains the same)

   c. HCO_3^- (_____ increases; _____ decreases; _____ remains the same)

   d. HCO_3^- to H_2CO_3 ratio (_____ increases; _____ decreases; _____ remains the same)

   e. pH (_____ increases; _____ decreases; _____ remains the same)

5. In **chronic alveolar hyperventilation**, the kidneys work to correct the pH status by:

   a. excreting HCO_3^-
   b. retaining H_2CO_3
   c. excreting H_2CO_3
   d. retaining HCO_3^-

6. In chronic alveolar hyperventilation, partial or complete renal compensation can be verified when the HCO_3^- and pH readings are:

   a. greater than expected for a particular Pa_{CO_2}
   b. less than expected for a particular Pa_{CO_2}

7. True _____ False _____ As a general rule, the kidneys have a tendency to overcompensate for an abnormal pH.

8. When **metabolic acidosis** is present, the HCO_3^- and pH readings are:

   a. greater than expected for a particular Pa_{CO_2}
   b. less than expected for a particular Pa_{CO_2}

9. List three common causes of metabolic acidosis:

a. ______________________________

b. ______________________________

c. ______________________________

10. In response to a metabolic acidosis condition, the ventilatory rate:

a. increases
b. decreases
c. remains the same

11. When **metabolic alkalosis** is present, the HCO_3^- and pH readings are:

a. greater than expected for a particular Pa_{CO_2}
b. less than expected for a particular Pa_{CO_2}

12. List five common causes of metabolic alkalosis:

a. ______________________________

b. ______________________________

c. ______________________________

d. ______________________________

e. ______________________________

13. Using the $P_{CO_2}/HCO_3^-/pH$ nomogram below, answer the next four questions (a–d):

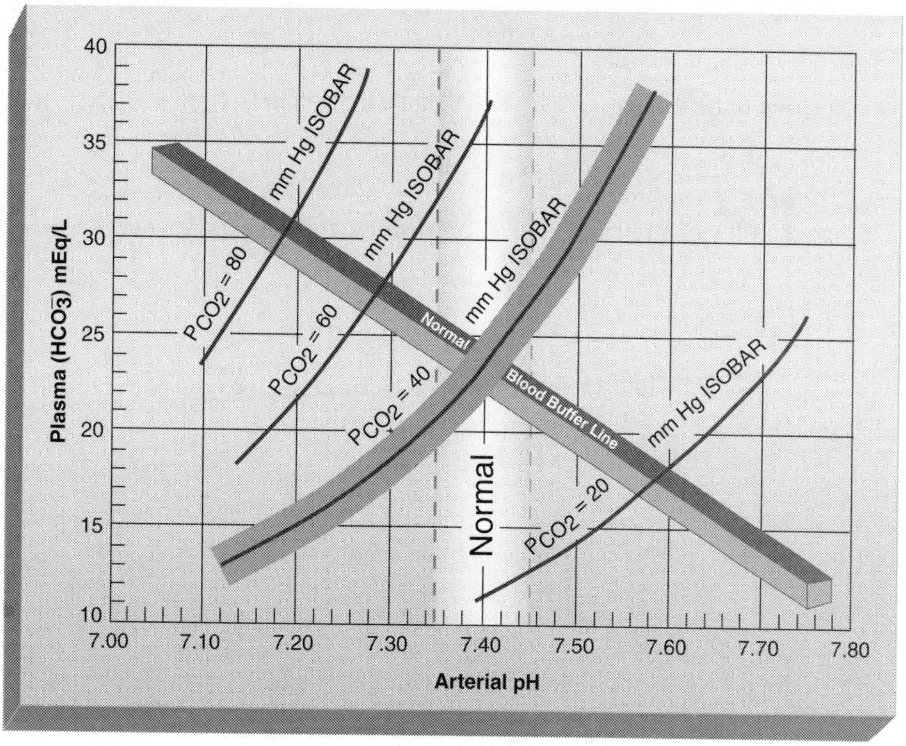

Figure 7–3 *Nomogram of $P_{CO_2}/HCO_3^-/pH$ relationship.*

a. If a patient's ventilatory rate suddenly decreased, and the patient's Pa_{CO_2} increased to 70 mm Hg, what changes would be expected in the pH and HCO_3^- level?

Answer: pH ______________________

HCO_3^- ______________________

b. If a patient's ventilatory rate suddenly increased, causing the patient's Pa_{CO_2} to decrease to 20 mm Hg, what would be the expected pH and HCO_3^- changes?

Answer: pH ______________________

HCO_3^- ______________________

c. If a patient presents with a pH of 7.2 and a Pa_{CO_2} of 60 mm Hg, does the patient have a metabolic or respiratory acid-base imbalance, or a combination of both?

Answer: ______________________________

Which does the above patient have, a base excess or a base deficit?

Answer: ______________________________

In order to return the patient's pH back to 7.4, how much of a base excess or base deficit does the patient have?

Answer: ______________________________

d. If a patient presents with a pH of 7.52 and a Pa_{CO_2} of 25 mm Hg, does the patient have a metabolic or respiratory acid-base imbalance, or a combination of both?

Answer: ______________________________

Which does the patient have, a base excess or a base deficit?

Answer: ______________________________

In order to return the patient's pH back to 7.4, how much of a base excess or base deficit does the patient have?

Answer: ______________________________

CHAPTER EIGHT

VENTILATION-PERFUSION RELATIONSHIPS

VENTILATION-PERFUSION RATIO

1. The normal alveolar ventilation is about ________ L/min.

2. The normal pulmonary capillary blood flow is about ________ L/min.

3. The average overall ventilation/perfusion ratio is ________ to ________, or ________.

4. In the normal individual in the upright position, the $\dot{V}/\dot{Q}$ ratio in the upper lung region is (_____ higher; _____ lower) than 0.8.

5. In the normal individual in the upright position, the $\dot{V}/\dot{Q}$ ratio in the lower lung region is (_____ higher; _____ lower) than 0.8.

6. In the upright lung, the $\dot{V}/\dot{Q}$ ratio progressively (_____ increases; _____ decreases; _____ remains the same) from the top to the bottom.

7. The $P_{A_{O_2}}$ is determined by the balance between

   a. ____

   ____

   b. ____

   ____

8. The $P_{A_{CO_2}}$ is determined by the balance between

a. ______________________________

____

b. ______________________________

____

9. When the $\dot{V}/\dot{Q}$ ratio increases, the $P_{A_{CO_2}}$ decreases because ______________________________

____

____

____

10. When the $\dot{V}/\dot{Q}$ ratio increases, the $P_{A_{O_2}}$ increases because ______________________________

____

____

____

____

11. In the upright lung, an increased $\dot{V}/\dot{Q}$ ratio is found in the:

a. upper lung regions
b. middle lung regions
c. lower lung regions

12. When the $\dot{V}/\dot{Q}$ ratio decreases, the $P_{A_{O_2}}$ decreases because ______________________________

____

____

____

13. When the $\dot{V}/\dot{Q}$ ratio decreases, the $P_{A_{CO_2}}$ increases because ______________________________

____

____

____

14. In the upright lung, a decreased $\dot{V}/\dot{Q}$ ratio is found in the:

   a. upper lung regions
   b. middle lung regions
   c. lower lung regions

15. In the upright lung, the Pc_{O_2} (_____ increases; _____ decreases; _____ remains the same) from the top to the bottom.

16. In the upright lung, the Pc_{CO_2}(_____ increases; _____ decreases; _____ remains the same) from the top to the bottom.

17. In the upright lung, the pH in the end-capillary blood (_____ increases; _____ decreases; _____ remains the same) from the top to the bottom.

18. **Internal respiration** is defined as ____

____

____

19. Normally, about __________ mL of oxygen are consumed by the tissue cells in 1 minute.

20. Normally, the tissue cells produce about __________ mL of carbon dioxide in 1 minute.

21. **Respiratory quotient** (RQ) is defined as the ____________________________________

____

____

22. The respiratory quotient is expressed as:

   RQ =

23. **External respiration** is defined as ____

____

____

24. **Respiratory exchange ratio** (RR) is defined as the ______________________________

____

____

25. List some pulmonary disorders that increase the $\dot{V}/\dot{Q}$ ratio:

a. ______________________________

____

b. ______________________________

____

c. ______________________________

____

d. ______________________________

____

e. ______________________________

____

26. List some pulmonary disorders that decrease the $\dot{V}/\dot{Q}$ ratio:

a. ______________________________

____

b. ______________________________

____

c. ______________________________

____

CHAPTER NINE

CONTROL OF VENTILATION

THE RESPIRATORY COMPONENTS OF THE MEDULLA

1. It is now believed that the DRG and VRG neurons in the medulla oblongata are responsible for coordinating the intrinsic rhythmicity of respiration. DRG and VRG are abbreviations for

   a. DRG: ______________________________

   a. VRG: ______________________________

2. The DRG consists chiefly of:

   a. inspiratory neurons
   b. expiratory neurons
   c. inspiratory and expiratory neurons

3. The VRG consists of:

   a. inspiratory neurons
   b. expiratory neurons
   c. inspiratory and expiratory neurons

4. Which of the following is activated only during heavy exercise or stress?

   a. DRG
   b. VRG

5. Where is the **apneustic center** located? ______________________________

6. If unrestrained, the apneustic center causes:
   a. prolonged expiration
   b. prolonged inspiration

7. Which of the following suppresses the function of the apneustic center?
   a. DRG
   b. pneumotaxic center
   c. VRG

MONITORING SYSTEMS THAT INFLUENCE THE RESPIRATORY COMPONENTS OF THE MEDULLA

1. The respiratory components (DRG and VRG) of the medulla are primarily influenced by an excessive concentration of __________.

2. Where are the **central chemoreceptors** located? __________

3. The **blood–brain barrier** is very permeable to __________ molecules, and relatively impermeable to __________ and __________ ions.

4. Write the chemical reaction that forms carbonic acid when CO_2 moves into the cerebrospinal fluid:

   $CO_2 +$

5. How do the central chemoreceptors respond to the liberated hydrogen ions [H+] produced in the above reaction?

6. In essence, the central chemoreceptors regulate ventilation through the (______ direct; ______ indirect) effects of CO_2 on the ________________________________.

7. The **peripheral chemoreceptors** are ________________________________

____

____

____

8. Where are the peripheral chemoreceptors located? ________________________________

____

____

____

9. When activated by a low Pa_{O_2}, the carotid bodies send neural impulses to the respiratory components of the medulla by way of the ________________________________ nerve; the aortic bodies send neural impulses to the medulla by way of the ________________________________ nerve.

10. Which of the following play a greater role in causing the ventilatory rate to increase in response to a decreased Pa_{O_2}?

    a. carotid bodies
    b. aortic bodies

11. At about what Pa_{O_2} level are the peripheral chemoreceptors significantly activated?

    Answer: ________________________

12. Suppression of the peripheral chemoreceptors is seen when the Pa_{O_2} falls below ________________ ________________________.

13. Why are the peripheral chemoreceptors totally responsible for the control of ventilation when the Pa_{CO_2} level is chronically high?

____

____

____

____

____

____

____

14. In response to a chronically high CO_2 level, the sensitivity of the peripheral chemoreceptors:

a. increases
b. decreases
c. remains the same

15. List some clinical conditions in which the P_{O_2} is normal, but the oxygen content is dangerously low:

a. ______________________________

b. ______________________________

c. ______________________________

16. List some other factors that stimulate the peripheral chemoreceptors:

a. ______________________________

b. ______________________________

c. ______________________________

d. ______________________________

e. ______________________________

17. In addition to an increase in ventilation, list some other responses that occur when the peripheral chemoreceptors are stimulated:

a. ______________________________

b. ______________________________

c. ______________________________

d. ______________________________

e. ______________________________

REFLEXES THAT INFLUENCE VENTILATION

1. What activates the **Hering-Breuer reflex?** ______________________________

____

2. When activated, the Hering-Breuer reflex cause(s) ______________________________

____

3. What activates the **deflation reflex?** ______________________________

____

4. When activated, the deflation reflex causes ______________________________

____

5. What activates the **irritant reflex?** ______________________________

____

____

6. Where are the irritant receptors located? ______________________________

____

7. When activated, the irritant reflex causes ______________________________

____

8. An extensive network of free nerve endings, called C-fibers, are located in the ____.

9. The C-fibers near the alveolar capillaries are called ________________.

10. The J-receptors are stimulated by ____.

11. When the J-receptors are stimulated, a reflex response triggers a ________________________.

12. **Peripheral proprioceptors** are located in the ________________________.

13. When stimulated, the proprioceptors send neural impulses to the ________________. The medulla, in turn, sends out an ________________________.

14. The proprioceptors in the joints and tendons are believed to play a role in initiating and maintaining an ________________________.

15. The more joints and tendons involved the ____________ the breathing rate.

16. Strong emotions can activate the centers in the hypothamus; for example, excitement causes the respiratory rate to (______ increase, ______ decrease).

17. An increased body temperature causes the respiratory rate to (______ increase, ______ decrease).

18. In response to an elevated systemic blood pressure, the **aortic and carotid sinus baroreceptors** cause ______________________________

____

19. In response to a reduced systemic blood pressure, the aortic and carotid sinus baroreceptors cause

____

____

CHAPTER TEN

FETAL DEVELOPMENT AND THE CARDIOPULMONARY SYSTEM

FETAL LUNG DEVELOPMENT

1. List the four periods of lung development during fetal life.

   a. ______________________________

   b. ______________________________

   c. ______________________________

   d. ______________________________

2. The lungs first appear as a small bud arising from the esophagus on the ____ day of embryonic life.

3. By the 16th week of gestation, there are about ____ generations of bronchial airways.

4. By the ____ week of gestation, the air–blood interface between the alveoli and the pulmonary capillaries and the quantity of pulmonary surfactant are usually sufficient to support life.

PLACENTA

1. Anatomically, the placenta consists of about 15 to 20 segments called ______________.

2. Label and color the following anatomic structures of the placenta:

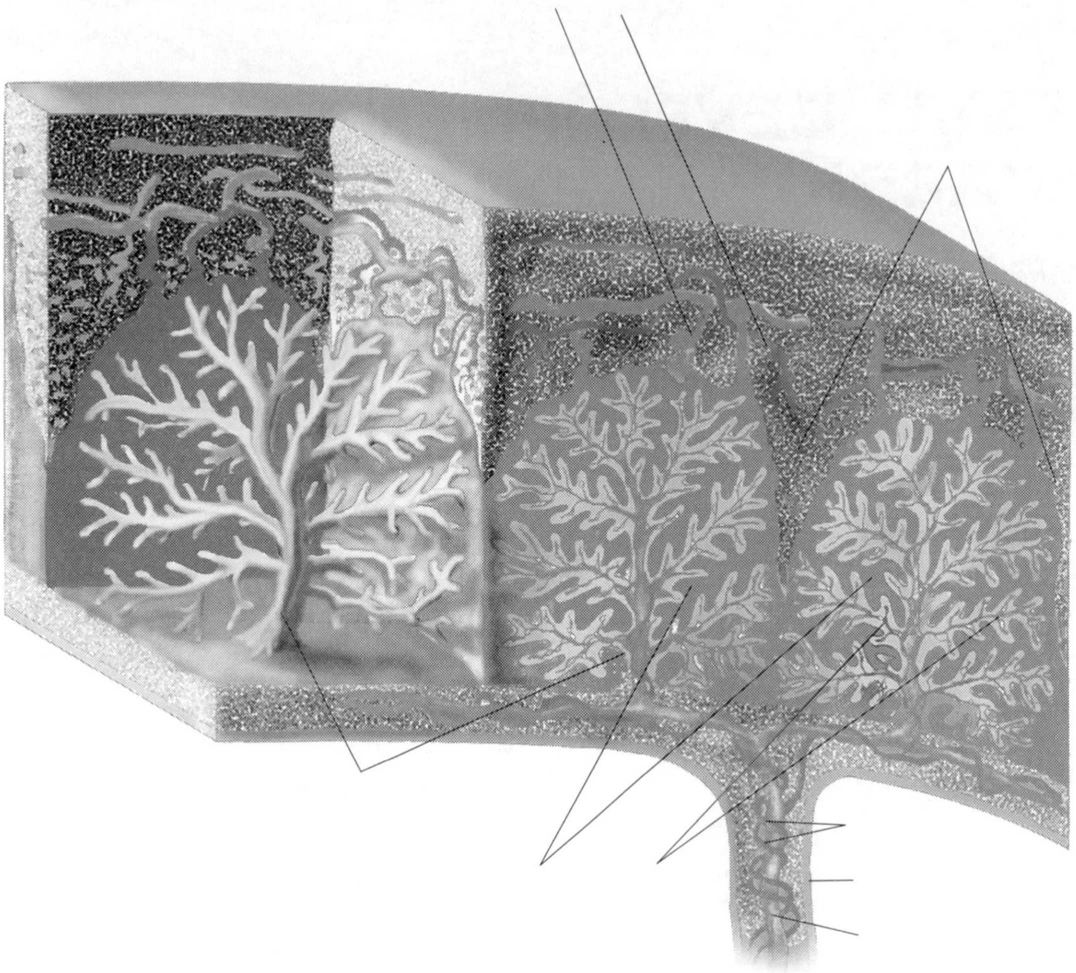

Figure 10–1 *Anatomic structure of the cotyledon of the placenta.*

3. Deoxygenated blood is carried from the fetus to the placenta by way of two ________________ ____.

4. Normally, the P_{O_2} in the umbilical arteries is about _____ mm Hg and the P_{CO_2} is about _____ mm Hg.

5. Explain why the maternal blood P_{CO_2} is frequently lower than expected during the last trimester of pregnancy.

____

____

____

____

6. Once in the intervillous space, oxygen transfers from the maternal to fetal blood because of the

a. ______________________________

____

b. ______________________________

____

c. ______________________________

____

7. As oxygenated fetal blood flows out of the chorionic villi, the P_{O_2} is about _____ mm Hg, and the P_{CO_2} is about _____ mm Hg.

8. Oxygenated fetal blood flows out of the chorionic villi and returns to the fetus by way of the _____ ______________________________.

9. List the three factors thought to be responsible for the wide variance between the maternal and fetal P_{O_2} and P_{CO_2}.

a. ______________________________

____

b. ______________________________

____

c. ______________________________

____

FETAL CIRCULATION

1. As oxygenated blood from the placenta returns to the fetus, about one-half of the blood enters the liver of the fetus and the rest enters the inferior vena cava by flowing through the ______________________________.

2. Once in the right atrium of the fetus, most of the blood flows directly into the left atrium through the ______________________________.

3. The blood in the left atrium of the fetus enters the ______________________________ and is then pumped primarily to the ______________ and ______________.

4. Most of the fetal blood that passes into the pulmonary artery from the right ventricle bypasses the lungs by passing through the ______________________________ and flows directly into the ______________________________.

5. Approximately ________ percent of the fetal circulation passes through the lungs and returns to the left atrium via the ______________________________.

6. The Pa_{O_2} in the descending aorta is about ____ mm Hg.

Matching:

7. Directions: In *Column A*, match the order (i.e., from first to last) in which fetal blood passes through the structures in *Column B*.

COLUMN A Order	COLUMN B Structure
_____	a. common iliac arteries
_____	b. external and internal iliacs
_____	c. ductus arteriosus
_____	d. umbilical arteries
_____	e. ductus venosus

8. Describe the changes the special structures of the fetal circulation go through after birth:

a. ______________________________

____

____

b. ______________________________

____

____

c. ______________________________

____

____

d. ______________________________

____

____

e. ______________________________

____

____

f. ______________________________

____

____

9. Describe the three primary mechanisms that remove the fluid from the fetal lungs during the first 24 hours of life:

   a. ______________________________

   ____

   ____

   b. ______________________________

   ____

   ____

   c. ______________________________

   ____

   ____

10. About ________ million primitive alveoli are present at birth.

11. The number of alveoli continues to increase until about ________ years of age.

BIRTH

1. List some of the stimuli that cause the infant to take its first breath at birth:

   a. ______________________________

   b. ______________________________

   c. ______________________________

2. During the first breath, it is estimated that the infant's intrapleural pressure decreases to about ________ cm H_2O before any air enters the lungs.

3. About ________ ml of air enters the lungs during the first breath.

4. The average lung compliance (C_L) of the newborn is about ________________.

5. The average airway resistance (R_{aw}) of the newborn is about ________________.

6. List the two major mechanisms that account for the decreased pulmonary vascular resistance when an infant inhales for the first time:

   a. ______________________________

   ____

   ____

   b. ______________________________

   ____

   ____

7. Describe the mechanism that causes the foramen ovale to close functionally at birth:

   ____

   ____

   ____

   ____

   ____

   ____

   ____

8. At birth, the newborn's P_{O_2} must increase to more than ______ to ______ mm Hg in order for the ductus arteriosus to close.

9. Describe the meaning of persistent pulmonary hypertension of the neonate (PPHN):

   ____

   ____

   ____

   ____

10. Persistent pulmonary hypertension of the neonate was previously known as ______________________________

    ______________________________.

11. List other substances that are released at birth that are believed to contribute to the constriction of the ductus arteriosus:

    a. ____________________

    b. ____________________

    c. ____________________

CONTROL OF VENTILATION IN THE NEWBORN

1. Although inhibited during fetal life, the ____________________ and ____________________ chemoreceptors play a major role in activating the first breath at birth.

2. Stimulation of the newborn's trigeminal nerve causes the infant's respiration and heart rate to ____________________.

3. Stimulation of the preterm infant's irritant reflex is commonly followed by ____________________.

4. Stimulation of the term infant's irritant reflex causes ____________________.

5. The head paradoxical reflex is: ____________________.

NORMAL CLINICAL PARAMETERS IN THE NEWBORN

1. Compare the approximate lung volumes and capacities of the newborn:

TABLE 10–1 Approximate Lung Volumes and Capacities of the Newborn

Tidal volume (V_T)	Vital capacity (VC)
Residual volume (RV)	Functional residual capacity (FRC)
Expiratory reserve volume (ERV)	Inspiratory capacity (IC)
Inspiratory reserve volume (IRV)	Total lung capacity (TLC)

2. Write the normal vital sign ranges of the newborn:

TABLE 10–2 Normal Vital Sign Ranges of the Newborn

Respiratory rate (RR)
Heart rate (HR)
Blood pressure (BP)

CHAPTER ELEVEN

AGING AND THE CARDIOPULMONARY SYSTEM

THE INFLUENCE OF AGING ON THE RESPIRATORY SYSTEM

1. The growth and development of the lungs is essentially complete by about ________ years of age.

2. Most of the pulmonary function indices reach their maximum level between ________ and ________ years of age.

3. With aging, the elastic recoil of the lungs (______ increases; ______ decreases; ______ remains the same), and the lung compliance (______ increases; ______ decreases; ______ remains the same),

4. With aging, identify which changes occur (check one) with the following lung volumes and capacities:

   a. RV (______ increases; ______ decreases; ______ remains the same)

   b. IC (______ increases; ______ decreases; ______ remains the same)

   c. IC (______ increases; ______ decreases; ______ remains the same)

   d. TLC (______ increases; ______ decreases; ______ remains the same)

   e. RV/TLC (______ increases; ______ decreases; ______ remains the same)

   f. FRC (______ increases; ______ decreases; ______ remains the same)

   g. ERV (______ increases; ______ decreases; ______ remains the same)

5. With aging, identify which changes occur with the following dynamic maneuvers of ventilation:

   a. FVC (_____ increases; _____ decreases; _____ remains the same)

   b. PEFR (_____ increases; _____ decreases; _____ remains the same)

   c. $FEF_{25\%-75\%}$ (_____ increases; _____ decreases; _____ remains the same)

   d. FEV_1 (_____ increases; _____ decreases; _____ remains the same)

   e. FEV_1/FVC ratio (_____ increases; _____ decreases; _____ remains the same)

   f. FRC (_____ increases; _____ decreases; _____ remains the same)

   g. MVV (_____ increases; _____ decreases; _____ remains the same)

6. With aging, identify which changes occur with the following components of the respiratory system:

   a. Pulmonary diffusing capacity (_____ increases; _____ decreases; _____ remains the same)

   b. Alveolar deadspace ventilation (_____ increases; _____ decreases; _____ remains the same)

   c. $P(A - a)_{O_2}$ (_____ increases; _____ decreases; _____ remains the same)

   d. Pa_{O_2} (_____ increases; _____ decreases; _____ remains the same)

   e. Pa_{CO_2} (_____ increases; _____ decreases; _____ remains the same)

   f. HCO_3^- (_____ increases; _____ decreases; _____ remains the same)

   g. pH (_____ increases; _____ decreases; _____ remains the same)

   h. $C(a - \bar{v})_{O_2}$ (_____ increases; _____ decreases; _____ remains the same)

   i. Hemoglobin concentration (_____ increases; _____ decreases; _____ remains the same)

ARTERIAL BLOOD GASES

1. With aging, the ventilatory response to both hypoxia and hypercapnia:

   a. increases
   b. decreases
   c. remains the same

2. With aging, the maximal oxygen uptake ($\dot{V}_{O_2}$ max):

   a. increases
   b. decreases
   c. remains the same

THE INFLUENCE OF AGING ON THE CARDIOVASCULAR SYSTEM

1. With aging, the elasticity of the heart:

   a. increases
   b. decreases
   c. remains the same

2. With aging, the work of the heart:

   a. increases
   b. decreases
   c. remains the same

3. With aging, the heart rate reacts as follows in response to stress:

   a. is more likely to increase dramatically
   b. is less likely to increase dramatically
   c. remains the same

4. What is the maximum heart rate for a 70-year-old?

   Answer: ______________________

5. With aging, identify which changes develop (check one) with the following components of the cardiovascular system:

   a. Stroke volume (_____ increases; _____ decreases; _____ remains the same)

   b. Cardiac output (_____ increases; _____ decreases; _____ remains the same)

   c. Resting pulse pressure (_____ increases; _____ decreases; _____ remains the same)

   d. Systolic blood pressure (_____ increases; _____ decreases; _____ remains the same)

   e. Peripheral vascular resistance (_____ increases; _____ decreases; _____ remains the same)

Section II

Advanced Cardiopulmonary Concepts and Related Areas—The Essentials

CHAPTER TWELVE

ELECTROPHYSIOLOGY OF THE HEART

ELECTROPHYSIOLOGY OF THE HEART

1. The way in which the heart contracts is by generating and propagating ____________________ ____________________________.

2. When the heart is relaxed (i.e., not generating an action potential), the cardiac muscle fibers are in what is called their __________________________ or _________________________.

3. When the heart is relaxed, there is an electrical charge difference across the fibers of the heart cells. This electrical difference between the electrolytes inside the cell membranes and the electrolytes outside of the cell membranes is called the ____.

4. The primary electrolytes responsible for the electrical difference across the RMP are ____.

5. When the heart is relaxed, the concentration of K^+ is (______ lowest, ______ greatest) inside the cardiac cell.

6. When the cardiac cell is relaxed, the inside of the cell is negatively charged with the ____________ and the outside of the cell is positively charged with the _______________________.

7. The RMP of the myocardial cells is about ________________________.

8. A cornerstone to the understanding of the electrophysiology of the heart are the five electrophysiologic phases of the ________________.

The Five Phases of The Action Potential

1. During Phase 0, an electrical impulse is initiated by the sinoatrial (SA) node. This action changes the RMP and allows a rapid inward flow of __________ into the cell through specific ______________. This process causes the inside of the cell to become ______________.

2. The voltage inside the cell at the end of depolarization is about __________. This electrophysiologic event produces a rapid (______ downstroke; ______ upstroke) in the action potential.

3. Immediately after phase 0, phase 1 starts. During this period the channels for __________ open and permit ______ to flow (____ in; ____ out) of the cell.

4. Phase 1 is illustrated as a short (____ downward; ____ upward) stroke in the action potential curve just before the plateau.

5. During this phase 2, there is a slow (____ inward; ____ outward) flow of ______, which in turn slows the (____ inward;____ outward) flow of ______ significantly.

6. During the plateau phase, the contraction of the myocardial cells are (____ prolonged; ____ shortened).

7. During phase 3, the (____ inward; ____ outward) flow of ______ stops, and the (____ inward; ____ outward) flow of ____ is again accelerated, and the rate of repolarization accelerates.

8. During phase 4, the excess ____ inside the cell and the loss of ____ are returned to normal by the ____ and ____ ion pumps.

PROPERTIES OF THE CARDIAC MUSCLE

1. The heart is composed of two types of cardiac cells: the ______________________ and the specialized "pacemaker cells" called the ______________________.

2. The myocardial ______________________ make up the bulk of the musculature of the myocardium, and are responsible for the pumping activity of the heart.

3. The majority of the autorhythmic cells are located in the ____________________.

4. **Automaticity** is the unique ability of the cells in the sinoatrial (SA) node (pacemaker cells) to generate an action potential without being stimulated. This is because the cell membranes of the pace maker cells permit Na^+ to leak (____ into; ____ out of) the cell during phase ____.

5. **Excitability** (irritability) is the ability of a cell to reach its threshold potential and respond to a stimulus or irritation. The lower the stimulus needed to activate a cell, the (____ less; ____ more) excitable the cell; the greater the stimulus needed, the (____ less; ____ more) excitable the cell.

6. **Conductivity** is the ability of the heart cells to ____________________ electrical current from ____________________ throughout the entire conductive system.

7. **Contractility** is the ability of cardiac muscle fibers to ____________________ in response to an electrical stimulus.

Refractory periods

1. The **absolute refractory period** is the phase in which the cells ____________________ ____________________.

2. Phase ____________________, represents the absolute refractory period.

3. The **relative refractory period** is the time in which repolarization is almost complete and a ____________________ stimulus may cause depolarization.

4. The second half of phase ____ represents the relative refractory period of the action potential.

5. The **nonrefractory period** occurs when all the cells are in their ____________________ ____________________.

6. Phase ____ represents the nonrefractory period.

The Conductive System

1. Using the following illustration, label the components of the conductive system of the heart:

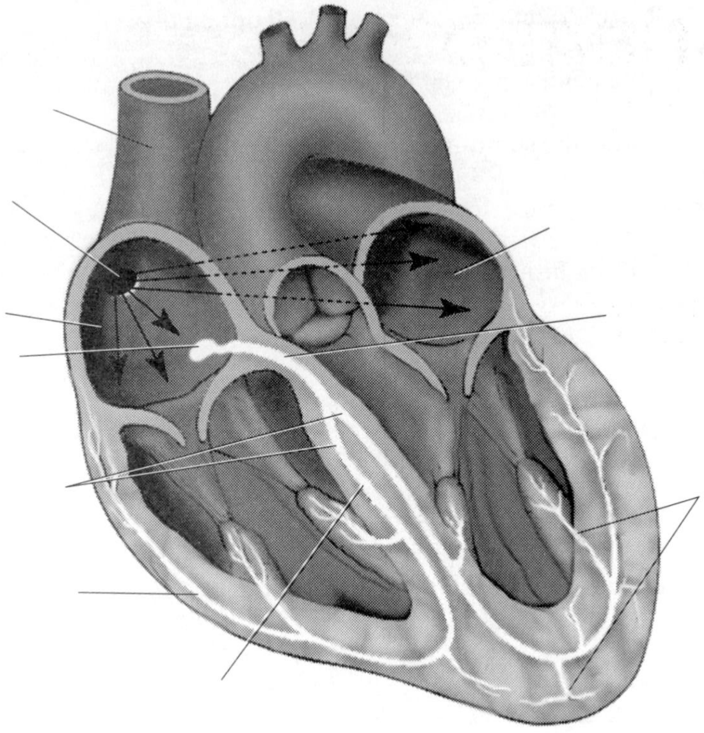

Figure 12–1 *Conductive system of the heart.*

Autonomic Nervous System

1. **Sympathetic** neural fibers innervate the atria and ventricles of the heart. When stimulated, the sympathetic fibers cause an *increase* in the ______________________________

______________________________.

2. Stimulation of the parasympathetic system causes a *decrease* in the ______________________________

______________________________.

CHAPTER THIRTEEN

THE STANDARD 12-ECG SYSTEM

THE STANDARD 12-ECG SYSTEM

1. The standard 12-ECG system consists of ______ limb electrodes and ______ chest electrodes.

2. In Table 13-1, list the 6 *standard limb leads* (bipolar and unipolar) and the 6 *precordial (chest) leads.*

Table13-1 ECG Lead Systems

STANDARD LIMB LEADS		PRECORDIAL (CHEST) LEADS
Bipolar Leads	Unipolar Leads	Unipolar Leads

3. Each lead:

a. ______________________________

b. ______________________________

c. ______________________________

Standard Limb Leads

1. Leads I, II, and III are ____________________, which means they use two electrodes to monitor the heart, one ______________ and one ______________.
2. An imaginary line, which can be drawn between the positive and negative electrodes for leads I, II, and III, represents the __________ of each lead.
3. The triangle formed around the heart by the three axes is called ____.
4. Electrical impulses that travel more toward the positive electrode (relative to the axis of the lead) are recorded as ____.
5. When an electrical current travels perpendicular to the lead axis, an ____________________ or ____________________ deflection is recorded.
6. Electrical impulses that move away from the positive electrode (or more toward the negative electrode) are recorded as ____________________ deflections in that lead.
7. In the normal heart, the largest electrical impulse travels from the _____ of the heart to the ____________, in a __________ to __________ direction.
8. Unipolar leads monitor the electrical activity of the heart between the __________ electrode and the __________ electrical reference point at the __________ of the heart. In essence, the __________ of the heart functions as a __________ electrode. Thus, the axis for these leads is drawn from the ______________ and the ______________ of the heart.
9. When the negative electrodes are eliminated in the aVR, aVL, and aVF, the amplitude of the ECG recordings are augmented by __________. This is the reason for the small case letter "a," which stands for ______________. The letter "V" represents ______________. The letters R, L, and F represent where the ____.

10. Collectively, the limb leads monitor the electrical activity of the heart in the ____________________, which is the electrical activity that flows over the anterior surface of the heart; from the ________________________________, in a __________ to __________ direction.

11. Leads I and aVL are called ______________________________, because they monitor the left lateral side of the heart. Leads II, III, and aVF view the lower surfaces of the heart and called the ____________________.

Precordial (Chest) Leads

1. The precordial leads monitor the heart from the ____________________, which means they record electrical activity that transverses through the heart. Leads V1 and V2 monitor the _________________________. V3 and V4 monitor the _________________________, and V5 and V6 view the ______________________________________.

2. Leads V1, V2, V3, and V4 are also called the ____________________. Leads V5 and V6 are also called the ______________________________________.

Modified Chest Lead

1. The *modified chest lead* (MCL_1) is a _______________ bipolar chest lead similar to the precordial lead. The positive electrode is on the chest and the negative electrode is on the ____.

NORMAL ECG CONFIGURATIONS AND THEIR EXPECTED MEASUREMENTS (LEAD II)

The ECG Paper

1. All ECG systems use the same standard paper and run at the same speed. Each **small square** has a duration of _______________ second. Each **large square**, delineated by the darker lines, has _______________ small squares, and a duration of _______________ second.

2. The paper on all ECG monitors run at a speed of ____________ large squares per second, or ____________ large squares per minute.

3. The vertical portion of each small square also represents an ____________ (or voltage) of ____________ **millivolt** (mV), and ____________ **millimeter** in distance.

4. Prior to each test, the ECG monitor is standardized so that 1 mV is equal to ____________ mm.

5. Most ECG paper has small vertical line marks in the margins every ____________ large squares, or every ____________ seconds.

6. A single *wave form* begins, and ends, at the ____________. When the wave form continues past the baseline, ____.

7. Two or more wave forms together are a ____________.

8. A flat, straight, or isoelectric line is called a ____________.

9. A wave form, or complex, connected to a segment is called an ____________

10. All ECG tracings above the baseline are described as ____________ deflections. Wave forms below the baseline are ____________ deflections.

The P-wave

1. The normal cycle of electrical activity in the heart begins with atrial depolarization and is recorded as the ____________.

2. The shape of the P-wave is usually ____________ and ____________.

3. The P-wave is followed by a short pause while the electrical current passes through the ____________.

4. This is seen on the ECG tracing as a ____________, or ____________, line after the P-wave.

5. The normal duration of the P-wave is ____________ to ____________ second, or ____________ small horizontal squares.

6. The normal amplitude of the P-wave is ____________ to ____________ mV, or ____________ small vertical squares.

7. An increased duration or amplitude of the P-wave indicates ________________.

8. Repolarization of the atria is usually not recorded on an ECG tracing. This is because atrial repolarization normally occurs when the ________________________________.

The P-R Interval

1. The *P-R interval* starts at the beginning of the ____________ and ends at the beginning of the ________________________________.

2. The normal duration of the P-R interval is ____________ to ____________ second, or ____________ to ____________ small horizontal squares.

3. The P-R interval represents the total atrial (supra-ventricular) electrical activity prior to the activation of the ____________, ____________, ________________ ________________________.

The QRS Complex

1. The *QRS complex* represents ________________________.

2. The QRS complex consists of three separate waves forms; the ____________, ____________, and ____________.

3. The first negative defection (below the baseline) after the P-wave is the ____________.

4. The next tall positive deflection (above the baseline) is the ____________.

5. The ________ wave is the small negative deflection (below the baseline) that follows the R wave.

6. Under normal conditions, the duration of the QRS complex is less than ____________ second, or ____________ small squares.

7. Abnormal ventricular-induced QRS complex waves are (_____ longer; _____ shorter) than _____ second.

8. Other characteristics of an abnormal QRS complex include ____________________, ____________________, and ____________________ ____________________.

The ST Segment

1. The *ST segment* represents the time between ____________________ and ____________________.
2. The ST segment begins at the end of the ____________________ and ends at the beginning of the ____________________.
3. Normally, the ST segment measures ______ second or less.
4. A flat, horizontal ST segment above or below the baseline is highly suggestive of ____________.

The T Wave

1. The *T wave* represents ____________________ ____________________.
2. Normally, the T wave has an positive deflection of about ________ mV.
3. The duration of the T wave normally measures ________ second or less.
4. At the beginning of the T wave, the ventricles are in their effective ____________________ ____________________.
5. At about the peak of the T wave, the ventricles are in their ____________________ period and, thus, are vulnerable to stimulation.
6. T waves are sensitive indicators for a number of abnormalities, including ____________________ ____________________ ____________________.

The U Wave

1. The *U wave* follows the ____________ and has the same polarity (deflection) as the ____________.

2. Because of its low voltage, the U wave usually is ____________.

The QT Interval

1. The *QT interval* is measured from the beginning of the ____________ to the end of the ____________.

2. The QT interval represents total ____________ ____________.

3. The normal QT measures about ________ second.

4. As a general rule, the QT interval should be about ________ of the measured R-R interval.

5. The QT interval varies ____________ to the heart rate.

CHAPTER FOURTEEN

ECG INTERPRETATION

STEP ONE: DOES THE GENERAL APPEARANCE OF THE ECG TRACING APPEAR NORMAL OR ABNORMAL?

1. Briefly describe how to assess the general appearance of an ECG for normal or abnormal tracings.

STEP TWO: DOES THE VENTRICULAR ACTIVITY (QRS COMPLEXES) APPEAR NORMAL OR ABNORMAL?

Rate

1. When the ventricular heart rate is **regular**, the rate can be determined by counting the number of ____________________ squares between two consecutive ____________________, and then dividing ____________________ by the number of ____________________ squares.
2. Complete the Estimated Heart Rate per Minute for Table 14-1 below:

TABLE 14-1 **Calculating Heart Rate by Counting the Number of Large ECG Squares**

DISTANCE BETWEEN TWO QRS COMPLEXES (NUMBER OF LARGE SQUARES)	ESTIMATED HEART RATE PER MINUTE
1	
2	
3	
4	
5	
6	

3. When the ventricular heart rate is **irregular**, the rate can be calculated by using the ____________________ in the upper margins of the ECG paper.
4. Calculating an irregular heart rate is done by counting the number of QRS complexes in a ____________________, and then multiplying this number by ____________________.

Rhythm

1. The ventricular rhythm is determined by comparing the ____________________ R-R interval with the ____________________ R-R interval.

2. When the time variation between the shortest R-R interval and the longest R-R interval is greater than ______________________ second, the rhythm is *irregular*.

Shape

1. The normal QRS duration is ______________ second or ______________.
2. A QRS complex that is narrow and 0.10 second or less represents a ______________________________.
3. When the QRS complex is greater than ______________ second, and the shape is ______________, an abnormal electrical source (ectopic focus) is likely to be present within the ventricle.

STEP THREE: DOES THE ATRIAL ACTIVITY APPEAR NORMAL OR ABNORMAL?

1. The **rate** of the atrial activity is calculated in the same way as the ______________________________.
2. Normally, the P-wave rate and the QRS rate are ______________.
3. The atrial **rhythm** is calculated in the same way as the ______________; except that in this case ______________ are used.
4. P-wave **shape** abnormalities may include ____.

STEP FOUR: DOES THE ATRIOVENTRICULAR RELATIONSHIP APPEAR NORMAL?

1. When the AV conduction ratio is greater than 1:1 (e.g., 2:1 or 3:1), not ____ ____________________ are being conducted to the ventricles.

2. The best method to determine the AV conduction ratio is to ask these two questions:

   a. ____

   b. ____

3. A P-R interval greater than ____________________ second represents an abnormal delay in AV conduction.

STEP FIVE: WHAT IS THE ECG INTERPRETATION?

1. Summarize the ECG characteristics of the normal sinus rhythm, as viewed from lead II, in the left side of the box below:

	Normal Sinus Rhythm
P-wave	
P-R Interval	
QRS Complex	
QRS Rate	
QRS Rhythm	

THE SINUS MECHANISMS

Sinus Bradycardia

1. *Bradycardia* means ______________________ heart.

2. In *sinus bradycardia*, the heart rate is less than ______________ beats per minute.

3. Summarize the ECG characteristics of the sinus bradycardia, as viewed from lead II, in the left side of the box below:

Sinus Bradycardia	
P-wave	
P-R Interval	
QRS Complex	
QRS Rate	
QRS Rhythm	

4. Common pathologic causes of sinus bradycardia include ______________________________

____

____

____

____.

5. Sinus bradycardia may lead to a ______________________________ cardiac output

and ______________________________________ blood pressure.

6. In severe cases, sinus bradycardia may lead to a ______________________________

perfusion and tissue ______________________________________.

Sinus Tachycardia

1. *Tachycardia* means ______________________________ heart.

2. In *sinus tachycardia*, the heart rate is between __________ and __________ beats per minute.

3. Summarize the ECG characteristics of the sinus tachycardia, as viewed from lead II, in the left side of the box below:

Sinus Tachycardia
P-wave
P-R Interval
QRS Complex
QRS Rate
QRS Rhythm

4. In the adult, sinus tachycardia is the normal physiologic response to ______________________________
____
______________________________.

5. Sinus tachycardia is also caused by physiologic stress such as ______________________________
____
____
______________________________.

6. Pathologic conditions associated with sinus tachycardia include ______________________________
____
____
______________________________.

Sinus Arrhythmia

1. In *sinus arrhythmia,* the heart rate varies by more than ______ percent.

2. The P-QRS-T pattern is (______ normal; ______ abnormal).

3. Summarize the ECG characteristics of the sinus arrhythmia, as viewed from lead II, in the left side of the box below:

Sinus Arrhythmia	
P-wave	
P-R Interval	
QRS Complex	
QRS Rate	
QRS Rhythm	

4. A sinus arrhythmia is a normal rhythm in ______________________________

   and ______________________________.

Sinus (SA) Block

1. In a *sinus (SA) block,* also called a ______________________________, the SA node initiates an impulse, but the electrical current through the atria is ______________________________.

2. When a sinus block occurs, the next P-QRS-T complex appears ______________________________

   ____

   ____

   ____

   ______________________________.

3. Summarize the ECG characteristics of the sinus (SA) block, as viewed from lead II, in the left side of the box below:

Sinus (SA) Block	
P-wave	
P-R Interval	
QRS Complex	
QRS Rate	
QRS Rhythm	

Sinus Arrest

1. *Sinus arrest* (SA node arrest) is the ______________________________________

____

____

______________________________________.

2. Summarize the ECG characteristics of the sinus arrest, as viewed from lead II, in the left side of the box below:

Sinus Arrest	
P-wave	
P-R Interval	
QRS Complex	
QRS Rate	
QRS Rhythm	

THE ATRIAL MECHANISMS

Premature Atrial Complex (PAC)

1. A *premature atrial complex* (PAC) results when ____

____

____

____.

2. Electrical currents that originate outside the SA node are called ______________________

____.

3. An ectopic foci in the atria results in a ______________________ on the ECG tracing.

4. Summarize the ECG characteristics of the premature atrial complex, as viewed from lead II, in the left side of the box below:

Premature Atrial Complex	
P-wave	
P-R Interval	
QRS Complex	
QRS Rate	
QRS Rhythm	

5. Causes of PACs include ____

____

____

____.

6. PACs are commonly seen in:

   a. ______________________________

   b. ______________________________

Atrial Bigeminy

1. *Atrial bigeminy* are said to be present is when ______________________________

   ______________________________.

2. Atrial bigeminy are often one of the first signs of ______________________________

   ______________________________.

Atrial Tachycardia

1. *Atrial tachycardia* is present when an atrial ectopic focus depolarizes the atria at a rate of

   ______________ to ______________ beats per minute.

2. When atrial tachycardia appears suddenly and then disappears moments later, it is referred to as

   ______________________________.

3. Summarize the ECG characteristics of atrial tachycardia, as viewed from lead II, in the left side of the box below:

	Atrial Tachycardia
P-wave	
P-R Interval	
QRS Complex	
QRS Rate	
QRS Rhythm	

4. Atrial tachycardia is associated with conditions that stimulate the sympathetic nervous system, such as ____
____
____.

Atrial Flutter

1. In *atrial flutter*, the normal P wave is absent and replaced by ______________________________
____.

2. Usually, the atrial rate is constant between ______ and ______ beats per minute while the ventricular rate is in the normal range.

3. Summarize the ECG characteristics of atrial flutter, as viewed from lead II, in the left side of the box below:

Atrial Flutter
ff Waves
P-R Interval
QRS Complex
QRS Rate
QRS Rhythm

4. Atrial flutter is frequently seen in patients over ______ years of age with ______________________
____
____
____.

Atrial Fibrillation

1. Atrial fibrillation is a chaotic ______________________________

____

____.

2. Atrial fibrillation is usually easy to identify and is often referred to as ______________

____.

3. The atrial rate cannot be measured, as it often reaches rates between ______________ and ______________ beats per minute.

4. The atrial P-waves are called ______________ or ______________.

5. Summarize the ECG characteristics of atrial fibrillation in the left side of the box below:

Atrial Fibrillation
ff Waves
P-R Interval
QRS Complex
QRS Rate
QRS Rhythm

6. Atrial fibrillation is associated with ______________________________

____

____

____.

7. Paroxysmal atrial fibrillation may also occur as a result of ______________________________

____

____.

THE VENTRICULAR MECHANISMS

Premature Ventricular Complex (PVC)

1. A *premature ventricular complex* (PVC) is the result of ______________________________

____

____.

2. Summarize the ECG characteristics of the premature ventricular complex in the left side of the box below:

Premature Ventricular Complex	
P-wave	
P-R Interval	
QRS Complex	
QRS Rate	
QRS Rhythm	

3. PVCs may occur in various forms, including ______________________________,

______________________________, ______________________________,

______________________________, and ______________________________.

4. *Uniform PVCs* (also called unifocal) orginate ______________________. All the PVCs on an ECG tracing are similar in ______________________.

5. *Multiform PVCs* (also called mutifocal) originate from ______________________ ______________________. When this occurs, the PVCs take on different ______________________.

6. *Paired PVCs* (also called couplets) are ______________________.

7. Ventricular *bigeminy* is a PVC ______________________ ______________________ ______________________.

8. *Trigeminy* is ______________________ ______________________.

9. Common causes of PVCs include ______________________ ______________________ ______________________ ______________________.

10. PVCs may also develop as a result of certain medications such as ______________________ ______________________ ______________________ ______________________.

Ventricular Tachycardia

1. Three or more PVCs occurring in a row represent ______________________ ______________________.

2. The rate is regular, or slightly irregular, between ______________ and ______________ beats per minute.

3. When ventricular tachycardia appears suddenly and then disappears moments later, it is referred to as ______________________ or ______________________ ventricular tachycardia.

4. When the ECG tracing shows only ventricular tachycardia, it is called______________________ ______________________ or ______________________.

5. The patient's blood pressure is often (_____ increased; _____ decreased) during ventricular tachycardia.

6. Summarize the ECG characteristics of ventricular tachycardia in the left side of the box below:

Ventricular Tachycardia	
P-wave	
P-R Interval	
QRS Complex	
QRS Rate	
QRS Rhythm	

Ventricular Flutter

1. In ventricular flutter, the QRS complex has the appearance of a ______________________ ______________________ ______________________ ______________________.

2. The rate is ______________________ to ______________________ beats per minute.

3. Summarize the ECG characteristics of ventricular flutter in the left side of the box below:

Ventricular Flutter	
P-wave	
P-R Interval	
QRS Complex	
QRS Rate	
QRS Rhythm	

Ventricular Fibrillation

1. *Ventricular fibrillation* is characterized by ______________________________

____

______________________________.

2. Ventricular fibrillation is a ______________________________ rhythm.

3. Summarize the ECG characteristics of ventricular fibrillation in the left side of the box below:

Ventricular Fibrillation	
P-wave	
P-R Interval	
QRS Complex	
QRS Rate	
QRS Rhythm	

Asystole (Cardiac Standstill)

1. *Asystole* is the ____

____

____.

2. The ECG tracing appears as ______________________________ and indicates

____

____

____.

AV CONDUCTION DEFECTS

Sinus Rhythm with First-degree AV Block

1. When the atrial impulse is delayed as it moves through the AV node, the P-R interval (__________ ______________________ increases; ______________________ decreases).

2. When the P-R interval is consistently greater than 0.20 second, a ______________________ ______________________________________ is said to exist.

3. Summarize the ECG characteristics of first-degree AV block, as viewed from lead II, in the left side of the box below:

First-degree AV Block
P-wave
P-R Interval
QRS Complex
QRS Rate
QRS Rhythm

4. Causes of first-degree AV blocks include ____

____

____.

Sinus Rhythm with Second-degree AV Block, The Wenckebach Phenomenon

1. The **Wenckebach** phenomenon is a ____

____

____

____.

2. Summarize the ECG characteristics of the Wenckebach in the space below:

____

____

____

____

____

____

____

Sinus Rhythm with Complete AV Block

1. When the pathology of the AV node is severe, all the sinus impulses may be ______________

____.

2. When a **complete AV block** is present, the ______________________________ takes control of the ventricular rhythm at a rate of ______________________________ to ______________________________ beats per minute. This mechanism is referred as the ____.

3. When the complete AV block is caused by pathology below the His bundle, the ventricular rhythm is controlled by what is called a ______________________________

____

______________________________.

4. The rate of the ventricular escape mechanism is between ______________

and ______________ beats per minute.

5. Summarize the ECG characteristics of complete AV block, as viewed from lead II, in the left side of the box below:

Complete AV Block
P-wave
P-R Interval
QRS Complex
QRS Rate
QRS Rhythm

CHAPTER FIFTEEN

HEMODYNAMIC MONITORING

HEMODYNAMIC MEASUREMENTS DIRECTLY OBTAINED BY MEANS OF THE PULMONARY ARTERY CATHETER

1. **Hemodynamic** is defined as ______________________________

____

____

2. Write the abbreviation and normal range for the following hemodynamic values directly obtained by means of the pulmonary artery catheter:

Table 15–1 **Hemodynamic Values Directly Obtained by Means of the Pulmonary Artery Catheter**

HEMODYNAMIC VALUE	ABBREVIATION	NORMAL RANGE
Central venous pressure		
Right atrial pressure		
Mean pulmonary artery pressure		
Pulmonary capillary wedge pressure (also called pulmonary artery wedge; pulmonary artery occlusion)		
Cardiac output		

HEMODYNAMIC VALUES COMPUTED FROM DIRECT MEASUREMENTS

1. Write the abbreviation and normal range for the following computed hemodynamic values:

Table 15–2 **Computed Hemodynamic Values**

HEMODYNAMIC VARIABLE	ABBREVIATION	NORMAL RANGE
Stroke volume		
Stroke volume index		
Cardiac index		
Right ventricular stroke work index		
Left ventricular stroke work index		
Pulmonary vascular resistance		
Systemic vascular resistance		

2. **Stroke volume** (SV) is defined as ______________________________

____

____

3. List the major determinants of stroke volume:

   a. ______________________________

   b. ______________________________

   c. ______________________________

4. Complete the following equation:

SV =

5. If a patient has a cardiac output of 5.5 L/min and a heart rate of 87 beats/min, what is the stroke volume?

Answer: ________________

6. The **stroke volume index** (SVI) is derived by________________

____

____

7. If a patient has a stroke volume of 55 ml and a body surface area of 2.5 m2, what is the SVI?

Answer: ________________

8. Clinically, what does the SVI reflect?

   a. ________________

   b. ________________

   c. ________________

9. The **cardiac index** (CI) is calculated by________________

____

____

10. If a patient has a cardiac output of 7 L/min and a body surface area of 2.5 m2, what is the CI?

Answer: ______________________

11. What does the **right ventricular stroke work index** (RVSWI) measure?

____

____

____

12. Clinically, what does the RVSWI reflect?

____

____

13. Complete the following equation:

RVSWI =

14. If a patient has a SVI of 40 ml, a $\overline{PA}$ of 25 mm Hg, and a CVP of 10 mm Hg, what is the RVSWI?

Answer: ______________________

15. What does the **left ventricular stroke work index** (LVSWI) measure?

____

____

____

16. Clinically, what does the LVSWI reflect?

____

____

17. Complete the following equation:

LVSWI =

18. If a patient has an SVI of 45 ml, an MAP of 125 mm Hg, and a PCWP of 10 mm Hg, what is the LVSWI?

Answer: ____________________

19. Fill in factors that increase and decrease the following hemodynamic variables:

Table 15–3 **Factors Increasing and Decreasing Stroke Volume (SV), Stroke Volume Index (SVI), Cardiac Output (CO), Cardiac Index (CI), Right Ventricular Stroke Work Index (RVSWI), and Left Ventricular Stroke Work Index (LVSWI)**

INCREASES	DECREASES
Positive Inotropic Drugs (Increased Contractility)	**Negative Inotropic Drugs (Decreased Contractility)**
Abnormal Conditions	**Abnormal Conditions**
	Hyperinflation of Lungs

20. The pulmonary vascular system is a (_____ high; _____ low) resistance system.

21. The systemic vascular system is a (_____ high; _____ low) resistance system.

22. Clinically, what does **pulmonary vascular resistance** (PVR) indicate?

Answer: ______________________________

23. Complete the following equation:

PVR =

24. If a patient has a $\overline{PA}$ of 20, a PCWP of 10 mm Hg, and a CO of 7 L/min, what is the PVR?

Answer: ____________________

25. Fill in under each category below the factors that increase pulmonary vascular resistance:

Table 15–4 Factors That Increase Pulmonary Vascular Resistance (PVR)

CHEMICAL STIMULI	**PATHOLOGIC FACTORS**
PHARMACOLOGIC AGENTS	
HYPERINFLATION OF LUNGS	
	HUMORAL SUBSTANCES

26. Fill in under the categories below factors that decrease pulmonary vascular resistance (PVR):

Table 15–5 Factors That Decrease Pulmonary Vascular Resistance (PVR)

PHARMACOLOGIC AGENTS	HUMORAL SUBSTANCES

27. Clinically, what does **systemic vascular resistance** (SVR) indicate?

Answer: ________________

28. Complete the following equation:

SVR =

29. If a patient has an MAP of 105 mm Hg, a CVP of 10 mm Hg, and a CO of 6 L/min, what is the SVR?

Answer: ________________

30. Fill in under the categories below factors that increase and decrease systemic vascular resistance (SVR):

Table 15–6 Factors That Increase and Decrease Systemic Vascular Resistance (SVR)

INCREASES	DECREASES
Vasoconstricting Agents	**Vasodilating Agents**
Abnormal Conditions	**Abnormal Conditions**

CHAPTER SIXTEEN

RENAL FAILURE AND ITS EFFECTS ON THE CARDIOPULMONARY SYSTEM

THE KIDNEYS

1. Label and color the following structures that form the **kidney**:

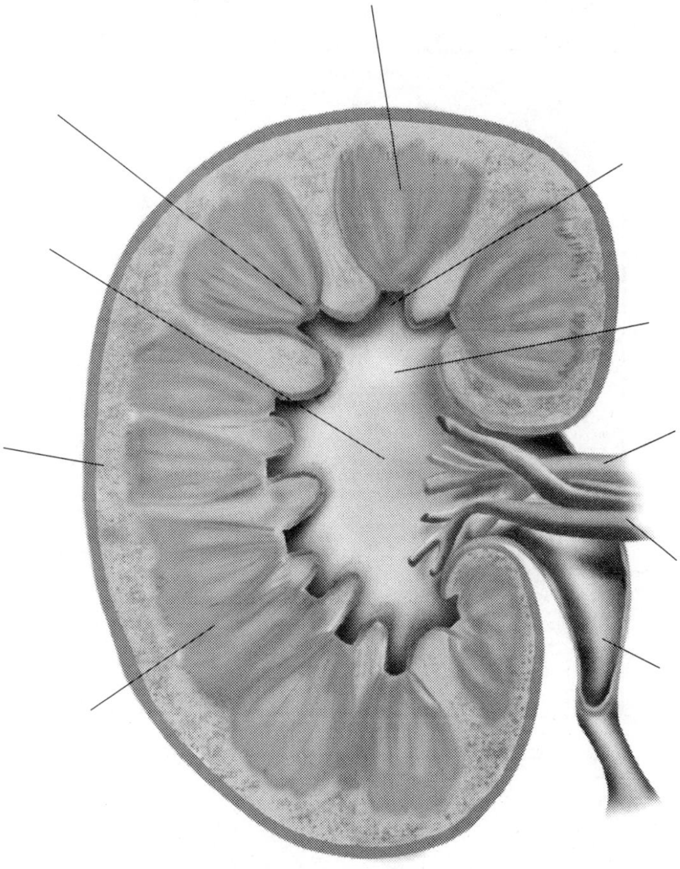

Figure 16–1 *Cross-section of the kidney.*

2. Label and color the following structures of the **nephron**:

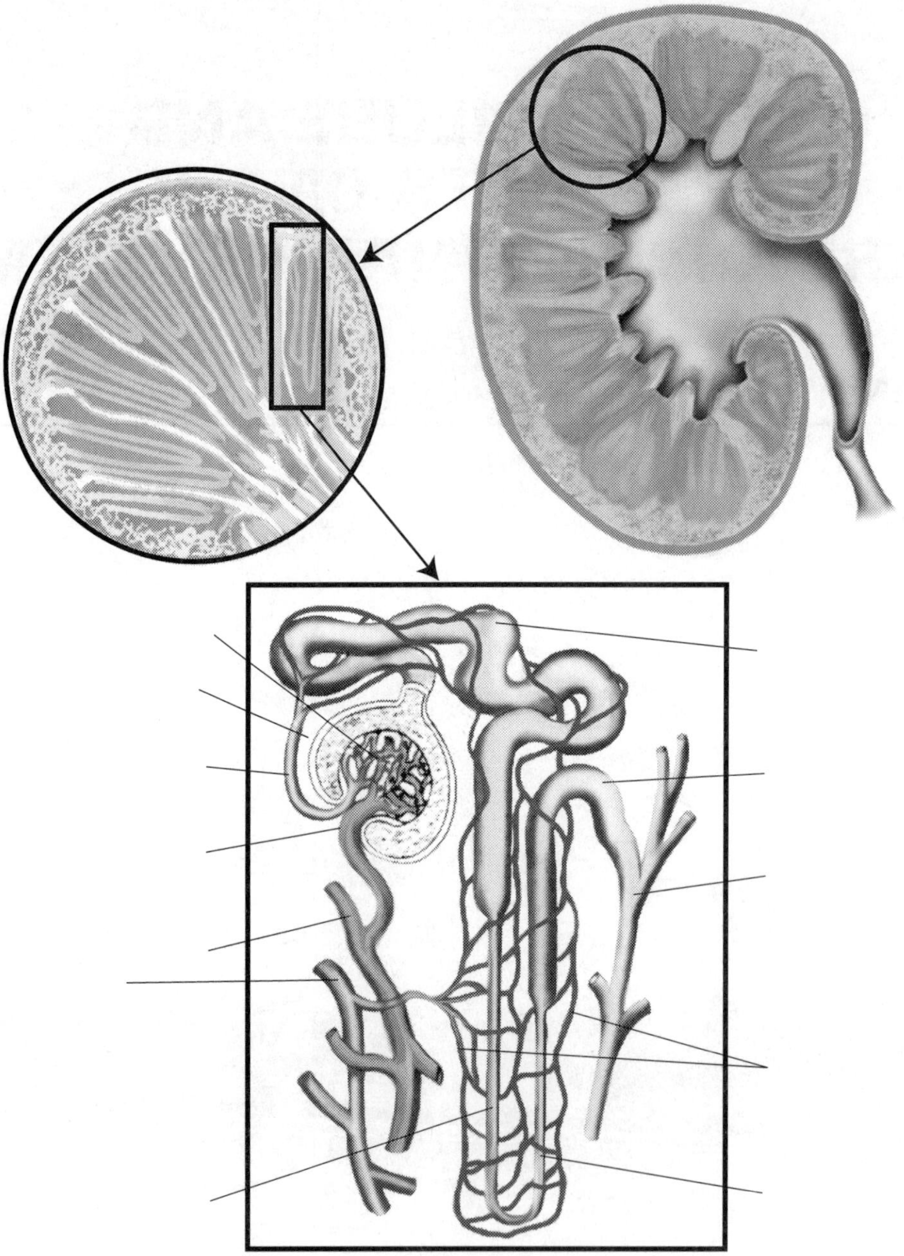

Figure 16–2 *The nephron.*

3. Label and color the following **blood vessels** of the kidney:

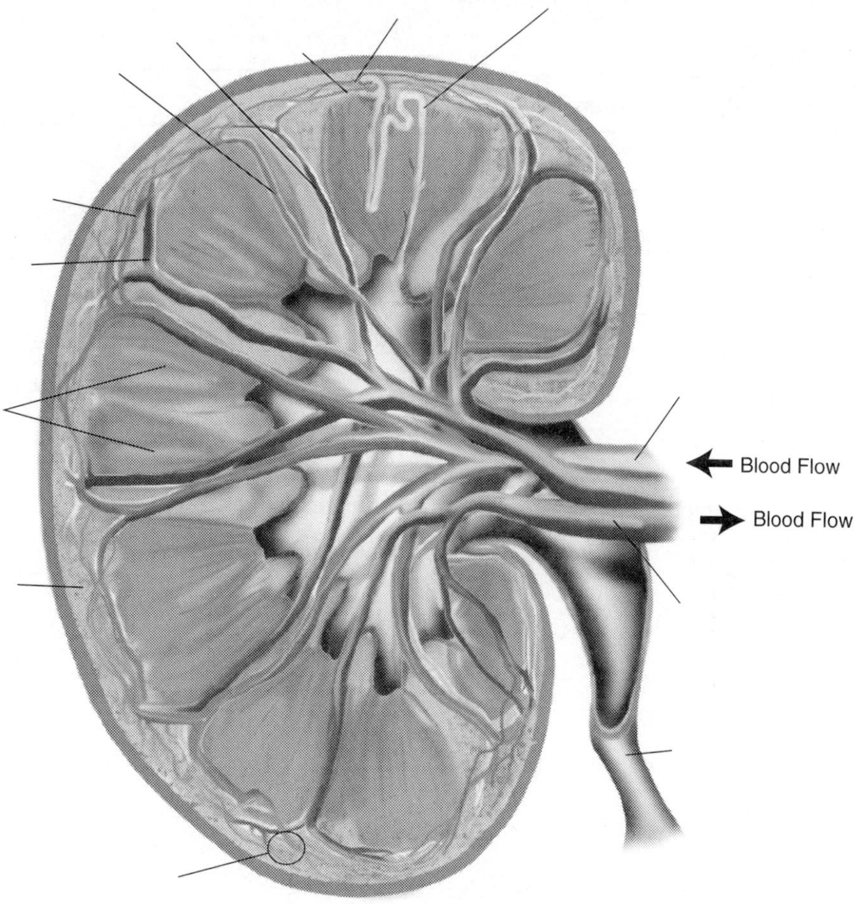

Figure 16–3 *Blood vessels of the kidney.*

URINE FORMATION

1. Compare the forces of glomerular filtration:

TABLE 16–1 Forces of Glomerular Filtration

FACTORS	FORCE
Enhances Filtration	
Glomerular capillary blood pressure	
Opposes Filtration	
Fluid pressure in Bowman's capsule	
Osmotic force (caused by the protein concentration difference)	________
Net Filtration Pressure	

2. List the three major structures responsible for tubular reabsorption:

   a. ________________________________

   b. ________________________________

   c. ________________________________

3. The bulk of **tubular reabsorption** occurs in the ________________________________

   ________________________________.

4. **Tubular secretion** is the mechanism by which ________________________________

   ____

   ____

   ____

   ____

5. The most important substances transported into the tubules by means of secretion are ________________ and ________________ ions.

URINE CONCENTRATION AND VOLUME

1. The kidneys control the concentration and volume of urine by virtue of the following two mechanisms:

   a. ______________________________

   b. ______________________________

   ____

2. The **juxtamedullary nephrons** are located deep into the ______________________________

   ______________________________.

3. The normal osmolality of the glomerular filtrate is approximately ________ mOsm/L.

4. The osmolality of the interstitial fluid ranges from about ________ mOsm/L in the cortex to about ________ mOsm/L as the juxtamedullary nephron descends into the renal medulla.

5. ADH is produced in the ______________________________ and released by the ______________________________.

6. When the atrial blood volume and pressure increase, the production of ADH:
   a. increases
   b. decreases
   c. remains the same

7. When the atrial blood volume and pressure decrease, the production of ADH:
   a. increases
   b. decreases
   c. remains the same

8. When the production of ADH decreases, the volume of urine (_____ increases; _____ decreases).

9. When the production of ADH increases, the volume of urine (_____ increases; _____ decreases).

10. The urine produced by the healthy kidney has a specific gravity of about ____________ to ____________.

REGULATION OF ELECTROLYTE CONCENTRATION

1. List some of the more important ions regulated by the kidneys:

   a. ______________________________

   b. ______________________________

   c. ______________________________

2. When the extracellular fluid becomes too acidic, the kidneys excrete ______________ ions into the urine.

3. When the extracellular fluid becomes too alkaline, the kidneys excrete (primarily) __________ ______________ into the urine.

4. The two major mechanisms responsible for maintaining an individual's blood volume at a consistent level are

   a. ______________________________

   b. ______________________________

RENAL FAILURE

1. List some congenital renal disorders:

   a. ______________________________

   b. ______________________________

   c. ______________________________

2. Urinary tract infections are seen more often in (_____ men; _____ women).

3. List some factors that predispose an individual to urinary flow obstruction:

   a. ______

   b. ______

   c. ______

   d. ______

   e. ______

4. List some causes of kidney inflammation:

   a. ______

   b. ______

   c. ______

5. Name the form of cancer that accounts for about 70 percent of all cancers of early childhood.

   Answer: ______.

6. List some common prerenal causes of renal failure:

   a. ______

   b. ______

   c. ______

   d. ______

7. What is one of the early clinical manifestations of **prerenal failure**?

   Answer: ______.

8. List the five categories of **renal** abnormalities that cause renal failure:

 a. ____________________

 b. ____________________

 c. ____________________

 d. ____________________

 e. ____________________

9. List some **postrenal** abnormalities that cause renal failure:

 a. ____________________

 b. ____________________

10. Positive pressure ventilation (____ increases; ____ decreases) urinary output.

11. Negative pressure ventilation (____ increases; ____ decreases) urinary output.

12. When positive pressure ventilation causes the blood volume and, therefore, the pressure in the atria to decrease, the release of ADH:

 a. increases
 b. decreases
 c. remains the same

13. When the concentration of ADH increases, the amount of urine formed:

 a. increases
 b. decreases
 c. remains the same

CARDIOPULMONARY PROBLEMS CAUSED BY RENAL FAILURE

1. Hypertension and edema develop in renal failure because of the kidney's inability to excrete ____________________.

2. When the kidneys fail, metabolic acidosis develops because the following changes occur:

a. H^+ (_____ increases; _____ decreases)

b. K^+ (_____ increases; _____ decreases)

c. HCO_3^- (_____ increases; _____ decreases)

3. **Hypochloremia** causes:

a. acidosis
b. alkalosis

4. **Hypokalemia** causes:

a. acidosis
b. alkalosis

5. **Hyperchloremia** causes:

a. acidosis
b. alkalosis

6. **Hyperkalemia** causes:

a. acidosis
b. alkalosis

7. Which two mechanisms contribute to the anemia seen in chronic renal failure?

a. ____

____

____

____

b. ____

____

____

____

8. Why do patients with chronic renal failure have a tendency to bleed?

9. Why is pericarditis seen in about 50 percent of persons with chronic renal failure?

Section III

THE CARDIOPULMONARY SYSTEM DURING UNUSUAL ENVIRONMENTAL CONDITIONS

CHAPTER SEVENTEEN

EXERCISE AND ITS EFFECTS ON THE CARDIOPULMONARY SYSTEM

EFFECTS OF EXERCISE

1. During heavy exercise

   a. Alveolar ventilation may increase as much as _____-fold.

   b. Oxygen diffusion capacity may increase as much as _____-fold.

   c. Cardiac output may increase as much as _____-fold.

   d. Muscle blood flow may increase as much as _____-fold.

   e. Oxygen consumption may increase as much as _____-fold.

   f. Heat production may increase as much as _____-fold.

2. Muscle training can increase muscle size and strength _____ to _____ percent.

3. The efficiency of intracellular metabolism may increase by _____ to _____ percent.

4. The size of the heart chambers and the heart mass of well-trained athletes may be increased by _____ percent.

5. The point at which anaerobic metabolism develops is called ______________________________.

VENTILATION

1. It has been suggested that the increased ventilation seen in exercise is caused by:

   a. ____

   ____

   ____

   b. ____

   ____

   ____

   c. ____

   ____

   ____

2. During strenuous exercise, an adult alveolar ventilation can increase to:

   a. 40 L/min
   b. 60 L/min
   c. 80 L/min
   d. 100 L/min
   e. 120 L/min

3. During exercise, the increased alveolar ventilation is caused mainly by an increased ________ of ventilation, rather than an increased ________ of ventilation.

4. During very heavy exercise, both an increased ________ and ______________ of ventilation are seen.

5. During very heavy exercise, the tidal volume is usually about what percent (circle one) of the vital capacity?

   a. 10%
   b. 20%
   c. 30%
   d. 40%
   e. 50%

6. There are three distinct consecutive breathing patterns seen during mild and moderate exercise.

   a. The first stage is characterized by ____________________

   ____

   ____

   ____

   b. The second stage is typified by ____________________

   ____

   ____

   ____

   c. During the third stage, ____________________

   ____

7. The maximum alveolar ventilation generated during heavy exercise under normal conditions is about ______ to ______ percent of the maximum voluntary ventilation.

8. At rest, normal oxygen consumption ($\dot{V}_{O_2}$) is about ______ mL per minute.

9. During exercise, the skeletal muscles may account for more than ______ percent of the ($\dot{V}_{O_2}$).

10. The Pa_{O_2} remains constant during:

    I. mild exercise
    II. moderate exercise
    III. heavy exercise

    a. I only
    b. I and II only
    c. I, II, and III

11. It has been shown that the increased oxygen diffusion capacity results from the ____________________ during exercise.

12. During exercise, the $P(A - a)_{O_2}$ remains essentially constant until what percent (circle one) of the maximal oxygen consumption is reached?

a. 10%
b. 20%
c. 30%
d. 40%
e. 50%

CIRCULATION

1. These essential physiologic responses must occur in order for the circulatory system to supply the working muscles with an adequate amount of blood:

a. ______________________________

b. ______________________________

c. ______________________________

2. The two circulatory effects of the sympathetic discharge are

a. ______________________________

____

____

____

b. ______________________________

____

____

____

3. The increased oxygen demands during exercise are met almost entirely by ______________________________

______________________________.

4. The increased cardiac output during exercise results from

   a. ______________________________

   b. ______________________________

   c. ______________________________

5. The increased stroke volume during exercise is primarily caused by ____________ in the working muscles.

6. The ability of the heart to accommodate the increased venous return and, subsequently, increase cardiac output is due to the ____________ curve.

7. The maximum heart rate for a 55-year-old is about ____________.

8. When the stroke volume decreases, the heart rate (____ increases; ____ decreases; ____ remains the same), and when the stroke volume increases, the heart rate (____ increases; ____ decreases; ____ remains the same).

9. The stroke volume is influenced by

   a. ______________________________

   ____

   b. ______________________________

   ____

   c. ______________________________

   ____

10. The body's ability to increase the heart rate and stroke volume during exercise progressively (____ increases; ____ decreases) with age.

11. There is almost always an increase in arterial blood pressure during exercise because of

a. ______________________________

____

____

b. ______________________________

____

____

c. ______________________________

____

____

12. As oxygen consumption and cardiac output increase during exercise, the pulmonary:

a. Systolic pressure (____ increases; ____ decreases; ____ remains the same)

b. Diastolic pressure (____ increases; ____ decreases; ____ remains the same)

c. Arterial (mean) pressure (____ increases; ____ decreases; ____ remains the same)

d. Wedge pressure (____ increases; ____ decreases; ____ remains the same)

13. The dilation of the blood vessels in the working muscles is caused primarily by ____________ ____________ acting on the arterioles.

STROKE VOLUME VERSUS HEART RATE IN INCREASING THE CARDIAC OUTPUT

1. During very heavy exercise, the increased ____________ accounts for a much greater proportion of the increased cardiac output than the ____________ .

2. The stroke volume reaches its maximum when the maximum cardiac output is only at approximately ____ percent.

3. After the stroke volume reaches its maximum, any further increase in cardiac output is solely caused by an ________________ .

4. Maximum exercise taxes the respiratory system only about _____ percent of maximum.

BODY TEMPERATURE/CUTANEOUS BLOOD FLOW RELATIONSHIP

1. List the symptoms that, collectively, are referred to as heat stroke:

____

____

____

____

____

____

2. The primary treatment of heat stroke consists of

   a. ____

   ____

   b. ____

   ____

   c. ____

   ____

   d. ____

   ____

CARDIOVASCULAR REHABILITATION

1. List the four phase(s) of the cardiovascular rehabilitation process:

   a. Phase I: ______________________________

   ____

   b. Phase II: ______________________________

   ____

   c. Phase III: ______________________________

   ____

   d. Phase IV: ______________________________

   ____

CHAPTER EIGHTEEN

HIGH ALTITUDE AND ITS EFFECTS ON THE CARDIOPULMONARY SYSTEM

EFFECTS OF HIGH ALTITUDE

1. The barometric pressure is about half the sea level value of 760 mm Hg at an altitude of ______ feet.

2. One of the most prominent features of acclimatization is ______________________________

____

3. In lowlanders who ascend to high altitudes, the RBCs increase for about ________ before the production rate levels off.

4. People who live at high altitudes commonly demonstrate:

   a. mild respiratory acidosis
   b. normal arterial blood gas values
   c. mild respiratory alkalosis

5. The oxygen diffusion capacity of lowlanders who are acclimatized to high altitude:

   a. increases
   b. decreases
   c. remains the same

6. The oxygen diffusion capacity of high-altitude natives is about ______________ than predicted.

7. At high altitude, the alveolar-arterial P_{O_2} difference $[P(A - a)_{O_2}]$:

   a. increases
   b. decreases
   c. remains the same

8. At high altitude, the overall ventilation-perfusion ratio improves in response to the (______ increased; ______ decreased) pulmonary arterial blood pressure.

9. In individuals who have acclimatized to high altitude, and in high-altitude natives, cardiac output:

   a. increases
   b. decreases
   c. remains the same

10. As an individual ascends, the pulmonary vascular system:

   a. constricts
   b. dilates
   c. remains the same

OTHER PHYSIOLOGIC CHANGES

1. In high-altitude natives, the concentration of myoglobin in skeletal muscles:

   a. increases
   b. decreases
   c. remains the same

2. Acute mountain sickness is characterized by ______________________________

   ____

   ____

   ____

3. The symptoms of acute mountain sickness are generally most severe on the ______________________________

   ____

   ____

4. Although the exact cause of high-altitude pulmonary edema is not fully understood, it may be associated with pulmonary (______ vasoconstriction; ______ vasodilation), and with a/an (______ increased; ______ decreased) permeability of the pulmonary capillaries.

5. High-altitude cerebral edema is characterized by________________________

____

____

____

6. Chronic mountain sickness is characterized by________________________

____

____

____

CHAPTER NINETEEN

HIGH-PRESSURE ENVIRONMENTS AND THEIR EFFECTS ON THE CARDIOPULMONARY SYSTEM

DIVING

1. For every 33 feet below the water surface, the pressure increases ______________________.

2. a. If an individual fully inhales to a total lung capacity of 5.5 liters at sea level, and dives to a depth of 99 feet, the lungs will be compressed to about:

   Answer: ______________________

   b. What is the pressure within the above diver's lungs?

   Answer: ______________________

3. The maximum time of a breath-hold dive is a function of

   a. ____

   ____

   b. ____

   ____

4. In regard to the P_{CO_2}, the so-called respiratory drive "breaking point" is about _____ mm Hg.

5. The so-called CO_2 paradox occurs as a diver (_____ descends; _____ ascends) and the O_2 paradox occurs as the diver (_____ descends; _____ ascends).

6. The fall in PA_{O_2} as a diver returns to the surface is known as the ______________________ ______________________.

7. The dive response consists of

   a. ____

   b. ____

   c. ____

8. List some of the signs and symptoms collectively referred to as decompression sickness:

   a. ____

   b. ____

   c. ____

   d. ____

   e. ____

HYPERBARIC MEDICINE

1. Identify indications for hyperbaric oxygenation for the following clinical conditions:

TABLE 19–1 **Indications for Hyperbaric Oxygenation**

GAS DISEASES
VASCULAR INSUFFICIENCY STATES
INFECTIONS
DEFECTS IN OXYGEN TRANSPORT

2. Hyperbaric oxygen is effective in the treatment of carbon monoxide poisoning. The administration of hyperbaric oxygen

a. ____

____

____

____

b. ____

____

____

____

c. ____

____

____

____

3. Breathing 100 percent oxygen at one atmosphere changes the CO_{Hb} half-life to less than ____________

____________________________.

ANSWERS TO CHAPTER EXERCISES

The question numbers refer to the questions in this workbook. The reference numbers refer to pages in the textbook, *Cardiopulmonary Anatomy and Physiology: Essentials for Respiratory Care*, Fourth edition.

CHAPTER ONE

THE ANATOMY AND PHYSIOLOGY OF THE RESPIRATORY SYSTEM

THE UPPER AIRWAY

1. (Fig. 1-1, pg. 8)
2. a. to act as a conductor of air
   b. to prevent foreign materials from entering the tracheobronchial tree
   c. to serve as an important area involved in speech and smell (ref. pg. 7)
3. a. filter
   b. humidify (ref. pg. 7)
   c. warm
4. (Fig. 1-2, pg. 9)
5. (Fig. 1-3, pg. 9)
6. pseudostratified ciliated columnar (ref. pg. 11)
7. a. superior nasal turbinates
   b. middle nasal turbinates
   c. inferior nasal turbinates (ref. pg. 11)
8. (Fig. 1-5, pg. 10)
9. levator veli platinum (ref. pg. 12)
10. stratified squamous (ref. pg. 8)
11. palatoglossal, palatopharyngeal (ref. pg. 12)
12. pseudostratified ciliated columnar (ref. pg. 13)
13. eustachian tube (ref. pg. 13)
14. stratified squamous (ref. pg. 12)
15. stratified squamous (ref. pg. 13)
16. (Fig.1-6, pg. 12)
17. a. acts as a passageway of air between the pharynx and the trachea
    b. works as a protective mechanism against the aspiration of solid and liquids
    c. generates sounds for speech (ref. pg. 12)
18. (Fig. 1-11, pg. 18)
19. (Fig. 1-7, pg. 14)
20. vocal ligament (ref. pg. 17)
21. thyroid cartilage (ref. pg. 17)
22. rima glottidis or glottis (ref. pg. 19)
23. stratified squamous (ref. pg. 13)
24. pseudostratified ciliated columnar (ref. pg. 13)
25. Valsalva's maneuver (ref. pg. 22)
26. (Fig. 1-13, pg. 20)
27. (Fig. 1-14, pg. 21)

THE LOWER AIRWAYS

The Tracheobronchial Tree

1. (Fig. 1-17, pg. 16)
2. a. epithelial lining
   b. lamina propria
   c. cartilaginous layer (ref. pg. 17)
3. pseudostratified ciliated columnar (ref. pg. 13)
4. submucosal glands (ref. pg. 24)
5. sol layer, gel layer (ref. pg. 25)
6. (Fig. 1-11, pg. 18)
7. a. cigarette smoke
   b. dehydration
   c. positive pressure ventilation
   d. endotracheal suctioning
   e. high inspired oxygen concentration
   f. hypoxia
   g. atmospheric pollutants
   h. general anesthetics
   i. parasympatholytics (ref. pg. 25)
8. a. histamine
   b. heparin
   c. slow-reacting substance of anaphylaxis
   d. platelet-activating factor
   e. eosinophilic chemotactic factors of anaphylaxis (ref. pg. 28)
9. 11 to 13, 1.5 to 2.5 (ref. pg. 28)
10. carina (ref. pg. 28)
11. 25, 40 to 60 (ref. pg. 29)
12. terminal bronchioles (ref. pg. 31)
13. increases (ref. pg. 32)
14. terminal bronchioles (ref. pg. 31)
15. mediastinal lymph nodes, the pulmonary nerves, muscular pulmonary arteries and veins, a portion of the esophagus, some visceral pleura (ref. pg. 33)
16. azygos, hemiazygos, intercostal veins (ref. pg. 33)
17. bronchopulmonary anastomoses (ref. pg. 34)

THE SITES OF GAS EXCHANGE

1. a. respiratory
   b. alveolar
   c. alveolar (ref. pg. 34)
2. (Fig. 1-25, pg. 19)
3. (Fig. 1-26, pg. 20)
4. 300 (ref. pg. 35)
5. 70 (ref. pg. 35)

6. respiratory bronchioles, alveolar ducts, and alveolar clusters (ref. pg. 34)
7. 130,000 (ref. pg. 35)
8. a. acinus
   b. terminal respiratory unit
   c. lung parenchyma
   d. functional units (ref. pg. 36)
9. squamous pneumocyte (ref. pg. 36)
10. granular pneumocyte (ref. pg. 36)
11. 95% (ref. pg. 36
12. Type II (ref. 36)
13. pores of Kohn (ref. pg. 36)
14. alveolar macrophages (ref. pg. 36)
15. tight space, loose space (ref. pgs. 36–37)

PULMONARY VASCULAR SYSTEM AND LYMPHATIC SYSTEM

1. (Fig. 1-29, pg. 39)
2. resistance (ref. pg. 40)
3. 0.1 μ, 10 μ (ref. pg. 40)
4. capacitance (ref. pg. 40)
5. visceral pleura (ref. pg. 41)
6. loose space of the interstitium (ref. pg. 41)
7. (Fig. 1-15, pg. 22)

NEURAL CONTROL OF THE LUNGS

1. autonomic nervous system (ref. pg. 43)
2. (ref. pg. 44)
3. epinephrine or norepinephrine (ref. pg. 43)
4. relax (ref. pg. 43)
5. constrict (ref. pg. 44)
6. acetylcholine (ref. pg. 44)

THE LUNGS

1. first (ref. pg. 44)
2. sixth, eleventh (ref. pg. 44)
3. hilum (ref. pg. 44)
4. costal, mediastinal (ref. pg. 44)
5. oblique fissure, fourth (ref. pg. 45)
6. costal, mediastinal (ref. pg. 45)
7. (Fig. 1-15, pg. 22)

8. (Fig. 1-34, pg. 45)
9. (Fig. 1-36, pg. 47)
10. (Fig. 1-37, pg. 48)

THE MEDIASTINUM, PLEURAL MEMBRANES, AND THORAX

1. trachea, heart, major blood vessels, various nerves, portions of the esophagus, thymus gland, and lymph nodes (ref. pg. 46)
2. visceral (ref. pg. 48)
3. parietal (ref. pg. 48)
4. pleural cavity (ref. pg. 48)
5. a. manubrium sterni
   b. the body
   c. xiphoid process (ref. pg. 49)
6. true ribs (ref. pg. 49)
7. false (ref. pg. 49)
8. floating (ref. pg. 49)
9. (Fig. 1-38, pg. 49)
10. (Fig. 1-39, pg. 50)

THE DIAPHRAGM

1. central tendon (ref. pg. 50)
2. esophagus, aorta, several nerves, and the inferior vena cava (ref. pg. 50)
3. phrenic (ref. pg. 50)
4. first, second (ref. pg. 52)
5. sternum (ref. pg. 52)
6. chest, anteroposterior (ref. pg. 53)
7. scapula, shoulders, arms (ref. pg. 54)
8. upward, outward (ref. pg. 55)
9. (Fig. 1-48, pg. 57)
10. downward, inward (ref. pg. 58)

CHAPTER TWO

VENTILATION

PRESSURE DIFFERENCES ACROSS THE LUNGS

1. driving pressure (ref. pg. 64)
2. transairway pressure (ref. pg. 65)
3. transpulmonary pressure (ref. pg. 65)
4. transthoracic pressure (ref. pg. 66)
5. 5 mm Hg (ref. pg. 65)
6. 7 mm Hg (ref. pg. 65)
7. 4 mm Hg (ref. pg. 65)
8. 6 mm Hg (ref. pg. 66)
9. decrease (ref. pg. 67)
10. greater (ref. pg. 67)
11. below (ref. pg. 68)
12. 3 to 6, 2 to 4 (ref. pg. 68)

STATIC CHARACTERISTICS OF THE LUNGS

1. study of matter at rest and the forces bringing about or maintaining equilibrium (ref. pg. 71)
2. collapse (ref. pg. 71)
3. expand (ref. pgs. 71)
4. a. the elastic properties of the lung tissue
   b. surface tension produced by the layer of fluid that lines the inside of the alveoli (ref. pg. 71)

ELASTIC PROPERTIES OF THE LUNGS

1. volume, pressure (ref. pg. 71)

Case A

2. a. (ref. pg. 71)
   0.055 L/cm H_2O (55 ml/cm H_2O)
   b. 0.070 L/cm H_2O (70 ml/cm H_2O)
   c. increasing

Case B

3. a. (ref. pgs. 71)
   0.050 L/cm H_2O (50 ml/cm H_2O)
   b. 0.045 L/cm H_2O (45 ml/cm H_2O)
   c. decreasing
4. 0.1 L/cm H_2O (ref. pg. 71)
5. 2,000 ml (2 liters) (ref. pg. 72)
6. right (ref. pg. 73)
7. a (ref. pg. 73)
8. b (ref. pg. 73)
9. the natural ability of matter to respond directly to force and to return to its original resting position or shape after the external force no longer exists (ref. pgs, 73–75)
10. the change in pressure per change in volume

    $$\text{Elastance} = \frac{\Delta P}{\Delta V} \quad \text{(ref. pg. 73)}$$

11. low, high (ref. pg. 73)
12. when a truly elastic body, like a spring, is acted on by 1 unit of force, the elastic body will stretch 1 unit of length, and when acted on by 2 units of force it will stretch 2 units of length, and so forth (ref. pg. 73)
13. volume, pressure (ref. pg. 75)
14. surface tension (ref. pg. 76)
15. 70 dynes/cm (ref. pg. 77)
16. $P = \frac{2ST}{r}$ (ref. pg. 77)
17. a. directly proportional to the surface tension of the liquid
    b. inversely proportional to the radius of the sphere (ref. pg. 77)
18. increases, decreases (ref. pg. 77)
19. b (ref. pg. 77)
20. critical opening pressure (ref. pg. 77)
21. c (ref. pg. 77)
22. alveolar Type II cells (ref. pg. 81)
23. water insoluble, water soluble (ref. pg. 81)
24. increases, decrease (ref. pg. 82
25. 5–15 dynes, 50 dynes (ref. pg. 84)
26. a. acidosis
    b hypoxia
    c. hyperoxia
    d. atelectasis
    e. pulmonary vascular congestion (ref. pg. 84)
27. low (ref. pg. 85)

DYNAMIC CHARACTERISTICS OF THE LUNGS

1. study of forces in action (ref. pg. 86)
2. the movement in action of gas in and out of the lungs and the pressure changes required to move the gas (ref. pg. 86).
3. $\dot{V} \approx \frac{\Delta P r^4 \pi}{81\eta}$ (ref. pg. 87)
4. a. increases
   b. increases
   c. increases
   d. increases (ref. pg. 87)
5. a. 2 liters/minute (L/min)
   b. 14 L/min
   c. 256 cm H_2O
   d. 20 cm H_2O
   e. 800 L/min
   f. 200 L/min
   g. 5 cm H_2O
   h. 2.5 cm H_2O (ref. pg. 87)
6. $\dot{V} \approx Pr^4$ (ref. pg. 88)

   $P \approx \frac{\dot{V}}{r^4}$ (ref. pg. 89)

AIRWAY RESISTANCE AND DYNAMIC COMPLIANCE

1. pressure difference between the mouth and the alveoli divided by flow rate (ref. pg. 90)
2. $R_{aw} = \frac{\Delta P(\text{cm } H_2O)}{\dot{V}(\text{L/sec})}$ (ref. pg. 90)
3. 3 cm H_2O/L/sec (ref. pg. 91)
4. 1.0, 2.0 (ref. pg. 91)
5. a gas flow that is streamlined (ref. pg. 92)
6. molecules that move through a tube in a random manner (ref. pg. 92)
7. time (in seconds) necessary to inflate a particular lung region to 60 percent of its potential filling capacity (ref. pg. 92)
8. b (ref. pg. 92)
9. b (ref. pg. 92)
10. c (ref. pg. 92)
11. a (ref. pg. 92)
12. a (ref. pg. 92)
13. e (ref. pg. 92)
14. change in the volume of the lungs divided by the change in the transpulmonary pressure during the time required for one breath (ref. pg. 93)

15. equal to (ref. pg. 94)
16. decreases (ref. pg. 94)
17. alveoli distal to an obstruction that do not have enough time to fill to their potential filling capacity as the breathing frequency increases (ref. pg. 94)

VENTILATORY PATTERNS

1. a. tidal volume
   b. ventilatory rate
   c. time relationship between inhalation and exhalation (ref. pg. 94)
2. 7 to 9, 3 to 4 (ref. pg. 94)
3. 15 (ref. pg. 94)
4. 1 : 2 (ref. pg. 94)
5. alveolar ventilation (ref. pg. 96)
6. deadspace ventilation (ref. pg. 96)
7. the volume of gas in the conducting airways: The nose, mouth, pharynx, larynx and lower airways down to, but not including, the respiratory bronchioles (ref. pg. 96)
8. 130 ml (ref. pg. 97)
9. tidal volume, deadspace ventilation, breaths per minute (ref. pg. 98)
10. 6,240 ml (ref. pg. 98)
11. an alveolus that is ventilated but not perfused with pulmonary blood (ref. pg. 99)
12. the sum of the anatomic deadspace and alveolar deadspace (ref. pg. 100)
13. greater (ref. pg. 100–101)
14. larger (ref. pg. 100–101)
15. c (ref. pg. 101)
16. increases, decreases (ref. pg. 101)
17. decreases, increases (ref. pg. 101)
18. energy, ventilation (ref. pg. 102)
19. complete absence of spontaneous ventilation (ref. pg. 103)
20. normal, spontaneous breathing (ref. pg. 103)
21. short episodes of rapid, uniformly deep inspirations, followed by 10 to 30 seconds of apnea (ref. pg. 103)
22. increased depth of breathing with or without an increased frequency (ref. pg. 103)
23. an increased alveolar ventilation produced by any ventilatory pattern that causes the $P_{A_{CO_2}}$ and, therefore, the Pa_{CO_2} to decrease (ref. pg. 104)
24. a decreased alveolar ventilation produced by any ventilatory pattern that causes the $P_{A_{CO_2}}$ and, therefore, the Pa_{CO_2} to increase (ref. pg. 104)
25. a rapid breathing rate (ref. pg. 104)
26. 10 to 30 seconds of apnea, followed by a gradual increase in the volume and frequency of breathing, followed by a gradual decrease in the volume of breathing until another period of apnea occurs (ref. pg. 104)
27. both an increased depth and rate of breathing (ref. pg. 105)
28. a condition in which an individual is able to breathe most comfortably in the upright position (ref. pg. 105)
29. difficulty in breathing, of which the individual is consciously aware (ref. pg. 105)

CHAPTER THREE

THE DIFFUSION OF PULMONARY GASES

DIFFUSION AND GAS LAWS

1. the movement of gas molecules from an area of relatively high concentration of gas to one of low concentration (ref. pg. 118)
2. if temperature remains constant, pressure will vary inversely to volume (ref. pg. 118)
3. $P_1 \times V_1 = P_2 \times V_2$ (ref. pg. 118)
4. 66.66 cm H_2O (ref. pg. 118)
5. 37.5 cm H_2O (ref. pg. 118)
6. if pressure remains constant, volume and temperature will vary directly (ref. pg. 119)
7. $V_1/T_1 = V_2/T_2$ (ref. pg. 119)
8. 9.37 L (ref. pg. 119)
9. 4.64 L (ref. pg. 119)
10. if the volume remains constant, pressure and temperature will vary directly (ref. pg. 119)
11. $P_1/T_1 = P_2/T_2$ (ref. pg. 119)
12. 156.2 cm H_2O (ref. pg. 119)
13. 44.53 cm H_2O (ref. pg. 119)
14. in a mixture of gases, the total pressure is equal to the sum of the partial pressures of each separate gas (ref. pg. 119)
15. 650 mm Hg (ref. pg. 119)

THE PARTIAL PRESSURES OF ATMOSPHERIC GASES

1. (ref. pg. 120)
2. decreases, remains the same (ref. pg. 121)
3. (ref. pg. 121)
4. the alveolar oxygen must mix—or compete, in terms of partial pressures—with alveolar CO_2 pressure and alveolar water vapor pressure (ref. pg. 121)
5. 44 mg/L, 47 mm Hg (ref. pg. 121)
6. 428.2 mm Hg (ref. pg. 122)

THE DIFFUSION OF PULMONARY GASES

1. a. liquid lining the intra-alveolar membrane
   b. alveolar epithelial cell
   c. basement membrane of the alveolar epithelial cell
   d. loose connective tissue (the interstitial space)
   e. basement membrane of the capillary endothelium
   f. capillary endothelium
   g. plasma in the capillary blood
   h. erythrocyte membrane
   i. intracellular fluid in the erythrocyte (ref. pg. 123)
2. 0.36 to 2.5 μ (ref. pg. 124)
3. 40, 46 (ref. pg. 124)
4. 60, 6 (ref. pg. 126)
5. 0.25 (ref. pg. 126)
6. 0.75, one-third (ref. pg. 126)
7. b (ref. pg. 127)
8. $\dot{V}\text{gas} \propto \frac{AD(P_1 - P_2)}{T}$ (ref. pg. 128)
9. a. a
   b. a
   c. b (ref. pg. 128)
10. the amount of gas that dissolves in a liquid at a given temperature is proportional to the partial pressure of the gas (ref. pg. 128)
11. solubility coefficient (ref. pg. 129)
12. a. directly proportional to the solubility coefficient of the gas
    b. inversely proportional to the square root of the gram-molecular weight of the gas (ref. pg. 129)

PERFUSION- AND DIFFUSION-LIMITED GAS FLOW

1. the transfer of gas across the alveolar wall is a function of the amount of blood that flows past the alveoli (ref. pg. 130)
2. the movement of gas across the alveolar wall is a function of the integrity of the alveolar-capillary membrane itself (ref. pg. 131)
3. a (ref. pg. 134)

CHAPTER FOUR

PULMONARY FUNCTION MEASUREMENTS

LUNG VOLUMES AND CAPACITIES

1. the volume of air that normally moves into and out of the lungs in one quiet breath. (ref. pg. 144)
2. the maximum volume of air that can be inhaled after a normal tidal volume inhalation. (ref. pg. 145)
3. the maximum volume of air that can be exhaled after a normal tidal volume exhalation. (ref. pg. 145)
4. the amount of air remaining in the lungs after a maximal exhalation. (ref. pg. 145)
5. the maximum volume of air that can be exhaled after a maximal inspiration. (ref. pg. 145)
6. the volume of air that can be inhaled after a normal exhalation. (ref. pg. 145)
7. the volume of air remaining in the lungs after a normal exhalation. (ref. pg. 145)
8. maximum amount of air that the lungs can accommodate. (ref. pg. 145)
9. the percentage of the TLC occupied by the RV. (ref. pg. 145)
10. (ref. pg. 145)
11. RV, V_T, FRC, RV/TLC ratio; VC, IC, IRV, ERV (ref. pg. 146)
12. VC, IC, RV, FRC, V_T, TLC (ref. pg. 146)
13. a. closed circuit helium dilution
    b. open circuit nitrogen washout
    c. body plethysmography (ref. pg. 146)

PULMONARY MECHANICS

1. the maximum volume of gas that can be exhaled as forcefully and rapidly as possible after a maximal inspiration. (ref. pg. 148)
2. the maximum volume of gas that can be exhaled within a specific period of time. (ref. pg. 149)
3. a. 60%
   b. 83%
   c. 94%
   d. 97% (ref. pg. 149)
4. decreases (ref. pg. 148)
5. comparison of the amount of air exhaled in 1 second to the total amount exhaled during a FVC maneuver. (ref. pg. 150)
6. Forced expiratory volume in 1 second percentage ($FEV_{1\%}$). (ref. pg. 150)
7. 83% (ref. pg. 150)
8. a. determine the severity of a patient's obstructive pulmonary disease
   b. distinguish between an obstructive and restrictive lung disorder (ref. pg. 150)

9. decreased (ref. pg. 150)
10. normal or increased (ref. pg. 150)
11. the average flow rate during the middle 50% of an FVC measurement. (ref. pg. 150)
12. medium, small (ref. pg. 150)
13. the average rate of airflow between 200 and 1,200 mL of the FVC. (ref. pg. 151)
14. large (ref. pg. 151)
15. the maximum flow rate that can be achieved. (ref. pg. 152)
16. the largest volume of gas that can be breathed voluntarily in and out of the lungs in 1 minute. (ref. pg. 154)
17. (Fig. 4-12, pg. 155)
18. (ref. pg. 157)

EFFECTS OF DYNAMIC COMPRESSION ON EXPIRATORY FLOW RATES

1. dependent on the amount of muscular effort exerted by the individual. (ref. pg. 157)
2. effort-dependent (ref. pg. 157)
3. once a maximum flow rate has been attained, the flow rate cannot be increased by further muscular effort (ref. pg. 157)
4. dynamic compression (ref. pg. 158)
5. toward the alveolus (upstream) (ref. pg. 158)
6. increases (ref. pg. 158)

CHAPTER FIVE

THE ANATOMY AND PHYSIOLOGY OF THE CIRCULATORY SYSTEM

BLOOD

1. a. plasma
   b. erythrocytes
   c. leukocytes
   d. thrombocytes (ref. pg. 170)
2. erythrocytes (ref. pg. 172)
3. 5 (ref. pg. 172)
4. 4 (ref. pg. 172)
5. hematocrit (ref. pg. 172)
6. a. 45%
   b. 42%
   c. 45 to 60% (ref. pg. 172)
7. 7.5 μ, 2.5 μ (ref. pg. 172)
8. 120 (ref. pg. 172)
9. Protect the body against the invasion of bacteria, viruses, parasites, toxins, and tumors. (ref. pg. 173)
10. 4000 to 11,000 (ref. pg. 173)
11. (ref. pg. 173)
12. neutrophils (ref. pg. 173)
13. eosinophils (ref. pg. 174)
14. Lymphocytes (ref. pg. 174)
15. Lymphocytes (ref. pg. 174)
16. platelets (ref. pg. 174)
17. 250,000 and 500,000 (ref. pg. 174)
18. prevent blood loss from a traumatized surface of the body involving the smallest vessels (ref. pg. 174)
19. 55 (ref. pg. 175)
20. 90 (ref. pg. 175)
21. a. albumins
    b. globulins
    c. fibrinogen (ref. pg. 175)
22. a. Na^+
    b. K^+
    c. Ca^{2+}
    d. Mg^{2+} (ref. pg. 175)

23. a. Cl^-
 b. PO_4^{3-}
 c. SO_4^{2-}
 d. HCO_3^- (ref. pg. 175)
24. a. amino acids
 b. glucose/carbohydrates
 c. lipids
 d. individual vitamins (ref. pg. 175)
25. a. urea
 b. creatinine
 c. uric acid
 d. bilirubin (ref. pg. 175)

THE HEART

1. (Fig. 5-2, pg. 176)
2. atria, ventricles (ref. pg. 175)
3. interatrial septum, interventricular septum (ref. pg. 175)
4. unoxygenated blood to the lungs (ref. pg. 177)
5. oxygenated blood throughout the systemic circulation (ref. pg. 177)
6. 250, 350 (ref. pg. 177)
7. point of maximal intensity (PMI) (ref. pg. 177)

The Pericardium

1. pericardium (ref. pg. 177)
2. a. protect the heart
 b. anchor it to surrounding structures, such as the diaphragm and the great vessels
 c. prevent the heart from overfilling (ref. pg. 177)
3. parietal layer, visceral layer (ref. pg. 177)

THE WALL OF THE HEART

1. a single sheet of squamous epithelial cells overlying delicate connective tissue (ref. pg. 177)
2. cross-striated tissue fibers that form a network of spiral bundles throughout the internal portion of the heart (ref. pg. 177)
3. inner myocardial surface; it lines the heart chambers (ref. pg. 179)

BLOOD SUPPLY OF THE HEART

1. left coronary artery, the right coronary artery (ref. pg. 180)
2. circumflex, anterior interventricular branches (ref. pg. 180)
3. marginal branch, posterior interventricular branch (ref. pg. 180)

4. great cardiac veins (ref. pg. 180)
5. middle cardia vein (ref. pg. 181)
6. coronary sinus (ref. pg. 181)
7. thebesian vein (ref. pg. 181)

BLOOD FLOW THROUGH THE HEART

1. inferior and superior vena cava (ref. pg. 181)
2. thebesian vein (ref. pg. 181)
3. tricuspid valve (ref. pg. 181)
4. chordae tendinae (ref. pg. 181)
5. papillary muscles (ref. pg. 182)
6. pulmonary trunk, pulmonary arteries (ref. pg. 182)
7. pulmonary semilunar valve (ref. pg. 182)
8. pulmonary veins (ref. pg. 182)
9. bicuspid valve (also called the mitral valve) (ref. pg. 182)
10. aorta (ref. pg. 182)

THE PULMONARY AND SYSTEMIC VASCULAR SYSTEMS

1. pulmonary trunk, left atrium (ref. pg. 183)
2. aorta, right atrium (ref. pg. 183)
3. away from (ref. pg. 183)
4. arterioles (ref. pg. 183)
5. arterioles (ref. pg. 183)
6. arterioles (ref. pg. 183)
7. external (ref. pg. 183)
8. internal (ref. pg. 183)
9. venules (ref. pg. 183)
10. capacitance (ref. pg. 183)
11. 60 (ref. pg. 183)
12. sympathetic (ref. pg. 183)
13. vasomotor, medulla oblongata, sympathetic (ref. pg. 183)
14. sympathetic (ref. pg. 183)
15. vasomotor tone (ref. pg. 183)
16. increasing, sympathetic (ref. pg. 183)
17. decreasing, sympathetic (ref. pg. 183)
18. a. heart
    b. brain
    c. skeletal muscles (ref. pg. 183)
19. pressoreceptors (ref. pg. 185)
20. glossopharyngeal (ref. pg. 185)
21. vagus (ref. pg. 185)
22. decrease, increase (ref. pg. 185)

23. a. an increased cardiac output
    b. an increase in the total peripheral resistance
    c. the return of blood pressure toward normal (ref. pg. 187)
24. a. large arteries
    b. large veins
    c. pulmonary vessels
    d. cardiac walls (ref. pg. 187)

PRESSURES IN THE PULMONARY AND SYSTEMIC VASCULAR SYSTEMS

1. actual blood pressure in the lumen of any vessel at any point relative to the barometric pressure (ref. pg. 187)
2. difference between the pressure in the lumen of a vessel and the pressure surrounding the vessel (ref. pg. 187)
3. greater than (ref. pg. 188)
4. less than (ref. pg. 188)
5. pressure difference between the pressure at one point in a vessel and the pressure at any other point downstream in the vessel (ref. pg. 188)

THE CARDIAC CYCLE AND ITS EFFECT ON BLOOD PRESSURE

1. systolic pressure (ref. pg. 188)
2. diastolic pressure (ref. pg. 188)
3. 10 (ref. pg. 190)
4. (Fig. 5-2, pg. 190)
5. 40 ml and 80 ml (ref. pg. 191)
6. cardiac output (ref. pg. 191)
7. 4,400 ml (ref. pg. 191)
8. a (ref. pg. 192)
9. 5 (ref. pg. 192)
10. 75, 15, 10 (ref. pg. 192)
11. 60, 10 (ref. pg. 192)

THE DISTRIBUTION OF PULMONARY BLOOD FLOW

1. to the portion of the body, or portion of the organ, that is closest to the ground (ref. pg. 192)
2. greater than (ref. pg. 193)
3. a. posterior
   b. anterior
   c. lung nearest the ground
   d. apices (ref. pg. 193)

4. greater than (ref. pg. 193)
5. a. severe hemorrhage
   b. dehydration
   c. positive pressure ventilation (ref. pg. 193)
6. alveolar dead space (ref. pg. 193)
7. greater than, greater than (ref. pg. 193)
8. greater than, less than (ref. pg. 194)
9. a. ventricular preload
   b. ventricular afterload
   c. myocardial contractility (ref. pg. 194)
10. the degree to which the myocardial fiber is stretched prior to contraction (ref. pg. 195)
11. more (ref. pg. 195)
12. ventricular end-diastolic pressure (ref. pg. 196)
13. ventricular end-diastolic volume (ref. pg. 196)
14. a (ref. pg. 196)
15. Frank-Starling curve (ref. pg. 196)
16. the force against which the ventricles must work to pump blood (ref. pg. 196)
17. a. the volume and viscosity of blood ejected
    b. peripheral vascular resistance
    c. total cross-sectional area of the vascular space into which blood is ejected (ref. pg. 196)
18. arterial systolic blood pressure (ref. pg. 196)
19. $BP = CO \times SVR$ (ref. pg. 197)
20. the force generated by the myocardium when the ventricular muscle fibers shorten (ref. pg. 197)
21. b (ref. pg. 197)
22. a. pulse
    b. blood pressure
    c. skin temperature
    d. serial hemodynamic measurements (ref. pg. 197)
23. positive inotropism (ref. pg. 197)
24. negative inotropism (ref. pg. 197)
25. $\text{Resistance} = \dfrac{\text{mean blood pressure}}{\text{cardiac output}}$ (ref. pg. 197)
26. a (ref. pg. 197)

ACTIVE MECHANISMS AFFECTING VASCULAR RESISTANCE

1. the physiologic, pharmacologic, or pathologic processes that have a direct effect on the vascular system (ref. pg. 197)
2. a (ref. pg. 197)
3. a (ref. pg. 198)
4. a (ref. pg. 198)
5. a (ref. pg. 198)

6. a. epinephrine (Adrenaline)
   b. norepinephrine (Levophed)
   c. dobutamine (Dobutrex)
   d. dopamine (Intropin)
   e. phenylephrine (Neo-synephrine) (ref. pg. 198)
7. a. oxygen
   b. isoproterenol (Isuprel)
   c. aminophylline
   d. calcium-blocking agents (ref. pg. 198)
8. a. vessel blockage or obstruction
   b. vessel wall diseases
   c. vessel destruction or obliteration
   d. vessel compression (ref. pg. 198)

PASSIVE MECHANISMS AFFECTING VASCULAR RESISTANCE

1. a secondary change in pulmonary vascular resistance that occurs in response to another mechanical change (ref. pg. 199)
2. b (ref. pg. 199)
3. the opening of vessels that were closed, the stretching or widening of vessels that were open (ref. pg. 200)
4. b (ref. pg. 200)
5. high (ref. pg. 200)
6. low (ref. pg. 200)
7. low (ref. pg. 201)
8. high (ref. pg. 201)
9. low (ref. pg. 202)
10. high (ref. pg. 202)
11. b (ref. pg. 202)
12. a (ref. pg. 203)

CHAPTER SIX

OXYGEN TRANSPORT

OXYGEN TRANSPORT

1. (ref. pg. 212)

BLOOD GAS VALUE	ARTERIAL	VENOUS
pH	7.35–7.45	7.30–7.40
P_{CO_2}	35–45 mm Hg	42–48 mm Hg
HCO_3^-	22–28 mEq/L	24–30 mEq/L
P_{O_2}	80–100 mm Hg	35–45 mm Hg

2. maintains its precise molecular structure and freely moves throughout the plasma in its normal gaseous state (ref. pg. 213)
3. dissolved O_2 (ref. pg. 213)
4. a. 0.15
   b. 0.15 vol% (ref. pg. 213)
5. the amount of O_2 in ml that is in 100 ml of blood (ref. pg. 213)
6. 280 (ref. pg. 213)
7. A (ref. pg. 213)
8. four (ref. pg. 213)
9. $Hb + O_2 \rightleftarrows Hb_{O_2}$ (ref. pg. 213)
10. 50, 25 (ref. pg. 214)
11. oxyhemoglobin (ref. pg. 214)
12. reduced hemoglobin or deoxyhemoglobin (ref. pg. 214)
13. directly (ref. pg. 214)
14. two identical α chains, each with 141 amino acids, and two identical β chains, each with 146 amino acids ($\alpha_2\beta_2$) (ref. pg. 214)
15. two α, two γ (ref. pg. 214)
16. methemoglobin (ref. pg. 214)
17. a. 14–16
    b. 12–15
    c. 14–20 (ref. pg. 214)
18. 33 (ref. pg. 215)
19. 1.34 (ref. pg. 215)
20. a. Thebesian venous drainage into the left atrium

b. bronchial venous drainage into the pulmonary veins
c. alveoli that are underventilated in proportion to pulmonary blood flow (ref. pg. 215)

21. **Case A**
a. 0.165
b. 14.807
c. 14.972
d. 149.72
e. 898.32 (ref. pg. 215)
Case B
a. 0.15
b. 19.296
c. 19.446
d. 194.46
e. 680.61
f. 12.135
g. 24.57 (ref. pg. 215)

OXYGEN DISSOCIATION CURVE

1. percentage, pressure (ref. pg. 216)
2. a. the hemoglobin has an excellent safety zone for the loading of oxygen in the lungs
   b. the diffusion of oxygen during the transit time hemoglobin is in the alveolar-capillary system is enhanced
   c. increasing the P_{O_2} beyond 100 mm Hg adds very little additional oxygen to the blood (ref. pg. 217)
3. a. P_{O_2} reductions below 60 mm Hg indicate a rapid decrease in the amount of oxygen bound to hemoglobin
   b. a large amount of oxygen is released from the hemoglobin for only a small decrease in P_{O_2} (ref. pg. 218)
4. a 85%
   b. 17 vol% (ref. pg. 217)
5. the partial pressure at which the hemoglobin is 50% saturated with oxygen (ref. pg. 218)
6. 27 (ref. pg. 218)
7. a (ref. pg. 218)
8. b (ref. pg. 218)
9. a. ↑ pH
   ↓ P_{CO_2}
   ↓ temperature
   ↓ DPG
   HbF
   CO_{Hb} (ref. pg. 218)
   b. ↓ pH
   ↑ P_{CO_2}
   ↑ temperature
   ↑ DPG (ref. pg. 218)
10. b (ref. pg. 222)

11. a (ref. pg. 222)
12. a (ref. pg. 222)
13. b (ref. pg. 222)

OXYGEN TRANSPORT STUDIES

1. a. total oxygen delivery
   b. arterial-venous oxygen content difference
   c. oxygen consumption
   d. oxygen extraction ratio
   e. mixed venous oxygen saturation
   f. pulmonary shunting (ref. pg. 229)
2. a. body's ability to oxygenate blood
   b. hemoglobin concentration
   c. cardiac output (ref. pg. 229)
3. $D_{O_2} = Q_T \times (Ca_{O_2} \times 10)$ (ref. pg. 229)
4. 420 ml O_2/min (ref. pg. 229)
5. a. decline in blood oxygenation
   b. decline in hemoglobin concentration
   c. decline in cardiac output (ref. pg. 229)
6. between the Ca_{O_2} and the $C\overline{v}_{O_2}$ (ref. pg. 229)
7. $C(a - \overline{v})_{O_2} = Ca_{O_2} - C\overline{v}_{O_2}$ (ref. pg. 230)
8. 4 vol% (ref. pg. 230)
9. a. decreased cardiac output
   b. periods of increased oxygen consumption
      1. exercise
      2. seizures
      3. shivering postoperative patient
      4. hyperthermia (ref. pg. 231)
10. a. increased cardiac output
    b. skeletal relaxation
    c. peripheral shunting
    d. certain poisons (cyanide)
    e. hypothermia (ref. pg. 231)
11. oxygen consumption, oxygen uptake (ref. pg. 231)
12. $\dot{V}_{O_2} = QT[C(a - \overline{v})_{O_2} \times 10]$ (ref. pg. 231)
13. 600 ml O_2/min (ref. pg. 231)
14. a. exercise
    b. seizures
    c. shivering in postoperative patient
    d. hyperthermia (ref. pg. 232)

15. a. skeletal relaxation
    b. peripheral shunting
    c. certain poisons (cyanide)
    d. hypothermia (ref. pg. 232)
16. body surface area (BSA) (ref. pg. 232)
17. 125, 165 (ref. pg. 232)
18. extracted by the peripheral tissues divided by the amount of oxygen delivered to the peripheral cells (ref. pg. 232)
19. a. oxygen coefficient ratio
    b. oxygen utilization ratio (ref. pg. 232)
20. $O_2ER = \frac{Ca_{O_2} - C\bar{v}_{O_2}}{CaO_2}$ (ref. pg. 232)
21. 25 (ref. pg. 232)
22. a. 50 (ref. pg. 232)
    b. 425, 425 (ref. pg. 232)
23. a. decreased cardiac output
    b. period of increased oxygen consumption
       1. exercise
       2. seizures
       3. shivering in postoperative patient
       4. hyperthermia
    c. anemia
    d. decreased arterial oxygenation (ref. pg. 233)
24. a. increased cardiac output
    b. peripheral shunting
    c. certain poisons (cyanide)
    d. hypothermia
    e. increased hemoglobin concentration
    f. increased arterial oxygenation (ref. pg. 233)
25. 75 (ref. pg. 234)
26. 65 (ref. pg. 234)
27. a. decreased cardiac output
    b. periods of increased oxygen consumption
       1. exercises
       2. seizures
       3. shivering in postoperative patient
       4. hyperthermia (ref. pg. 234)
28. a (ref. pg. 234)
29. a. increased cardiac output
    b. skeletal relaxation
    c. peripheral shunting
    d. certain poisons (cyanide)
    e. hypothermia (ref. pg. 234)
30. b (ref. pg. 234)
31. (ref. pg. 235)

MECHANISMS OF PULMONARY SHUNTING

1. that portion of the cardiac output that enters the left side of the heart without exchanging gases with the alveolar gases—or the blood that does exchange gases with alveolar gases but does not obtain a P_{O_2} that equals the alveolus (ref. pg. 234)
2. a. anatomic shunts
   b. capillary shunts (ref. pg. 235)
3. blood flows from the right side of the heart to the left side without coming in contact with an alveolus for gas exchange (ref. pg. 235)
4. 2, 5 (ref. pg. 235)
5. a. congenital heart disease
   b. intrapulmonary fistula
   c. vascular lung tumors (ref. pg. 235)
6. a. alveolar collapse or atelectasis
   b. alveolar fluid accumulation
   c. alveolar consolidation (ref. pg. 237)
7. true, absolute shunt (ref. pg. 237)
8. The hypoxemia produced by an absolute shunt cannot be treated by simply increasing the concentration of inspired oxygen, as the alveoli are unable to accommodate any form of ventilation (ref. pg. 237)
9. pulmonary capillary perfusion is in excess of alveolar ventilation (ref. pg. 237)
10. a. hypoventilation
    b. uneven distribution of ventilation
    c. alveolar-capillary diffusion defects (ref. pg. 237)
11. the mixing of shunted, non-reoxygenated blood with reoxygenated blood distal to the alveoli (ref. pg. 237)
12. $\frac{\dot{Q}_S}{\dot{Q}_T} = \frac{Cc_{O_2} - Ca_{O_2}}{Cc_{O_2} - C\bar{v}_{O_2}}$ (ref. pg. 238)
13. a. 268.1 mm Hg
    b. 14.204 vol% $_{O_2}$
    c. 12.389 vol% $_{O_2}$
    d. 8.139 vol% $_{O_2}$
    e. 0.29 (ref. pg. 238)
14. a. reflects normal lung status
    b. reflects an intrapulmonary abnormality
    c. reflects significant intrapulmonary disease, and may be life-threatening in patients with limited cardiovascular or central nervous system function
    d. reflects a potentially life-threatening situation—aggressive cardiopulmonary support is generally required (ref. pg. 240)
15. a. questionable perfusion status
    b. decreased myocardial reserve
    c. unstable oxygen consumption demand (ref. pg. 240)

TISSUE HYPOXIA

1. the condition in which the Pa_{O_2} and Ca_{O_2} are abnormally low (ref. pg. 241)
2. a. low alveolar P_{O_2}
   b. diffusion impairment
   c. ventilation/perfusion mismatch (ref. pg. 241)
3. a condition in which the oxygen tension in the arterial blood is normal, but the oxygen-carrying capacity of the blood is inadequate (ref. pg. 241)
4. a. low amount of hemoglobin in the blood
   b. deficiency in the ability for hemoglobin to carry oxygen (ref. pg. 241)
5. a condition in which the arterial blood that reaches the tissue cells may have a normal oxygen tension and content, but the blood is not adequate to meet tissue needs (ref. pg. 242)
6. a. stagnant hypoxia
   b. arterial-venous shunting (ref. pg. 242)
7. any condition that impairs the ability of tissue cells to utilize oxygen (ref. pg. 242)
8. the term used to describe the blue-gray or purplish discoloration seen on the mucous membranes, fingertips, and toes (ref. pg. 242)
9. an increased level of red blood cells (ref. pg. 243)

CHAPTER SEVEN

CARBON DIOXIDE TRANSPORT AND ACID-BASE BALANCE

CARBON DIOXIDE TRANSPORT

1. a. carbamino compound
   b. bicarbonate
   c. dissolved CO_2 (ref. pg. 252)
2. a. dissolved CO_2
   b. carbamino-Hb
   c. bicarbonate (ref. pg. 253)
3. bicarbonate (ref. pg. 254)
4. 63 (ref. pg. 254)
5. (ref. pg. 253)
6. linear (ref. pg. 256)

CARBON DIOXIDE ELIMINATION AT THE LUNGS

1. 40, 50 (ref. pg. 256)

CARBON DIOXIDE DISSOCIATION CURVE AND ACID-BASE BALANCE

1. Haldane effect (ref. pg. 256)
2. charged species (ions) that can conduct a current in solution (ref. pg. 259)
3. substance that is capable of neutralizing both acids and bases without causing an appreciable change in the original pH (ref. pg. 259)
4. dissociates completely into H^+ and an anion (ref. pg. 259)
5. dissociates only partially into ions (ref. pg. 259)
6. dissociates completely (ref. pg. 259)
7. reacts with water to form OH^- in an equilibrium; partial dissociation (ref. pg. 259)
8. weak acid or base systems that have an equilibrium between the molecular form and its ions (ref. pg. 259)
9. $[H^+] + [A^-]$ (ref. pg. 259)
10. neutral (ref. pg. 259)
11. acidic (ref. pg. 259)

12. basic (ref. pg. 259)
13. the negative logarithm, to the base 10, of the hydrogen ion concentration (ref. pg. 259)
14. $pH = -\log_{10}[H^+]$ (ref. pg. 259)
15. 10^{-7} (ref. pg. 259)
16. donates (ref. pg. 259)
17. decreases (ref. pg. 259)
18. accepts (ref. pg. 259)
19. increases (ref. pg. 259)
20. a. the buffer systems of the blood and tissue
    b. the respiratory ability to regulate the elimination of CO_2
    c. the renal ability to regulate the excretion of hydrogen and reabsorption of bicarbonate ions (ref. pg. 259)
21. carbonic acid/sodium bicarbonate (ref. pg. 260)
22. $pK + \log \dfrac{[HCO_3^-]}{[H_2CO_3]}$ (ref. pg. 260)
23. the dissociation constant of the acid portion of the buffer combination (ref. pg. 260)
24. 6.1 (ref. pg. 260)
25. 20, 1 (ref. pg. 261)
26. b (ref. pg. 261)
27. c (ref. pg. 261)

THE ROLE OF THE P_{CO_2}/HCO_3^- pH RELATIONSHIP IN ACID-BASE BALANCE

1. a. increases
   b increases
   c. increases
   d. decreases
   e. decreases (ref. pg. 262)
2. d (ref. pg. 262)
3. a (ref. pg. 262)
4. a. decreases
   b. decreases
   c. decreases
   d. increases
   e. increases (ref. pg. 263)
5. a (ref. pg. 265)
6. b (ref. pg. 265)
7. False (ref. pg. 265)
8. b (ref. pg. 266)
9. a. lactic acidosis
   b. ketoacidosis
   c. renal failure (ref. pg. 266)

10. a (ref. pg. 266)
11. a (ref. pg. 267)
12. a. hypokalemia
    b. hypochloremia
    c. gastric suction or vomiting
    d. excessive administration of corticosteroids
    e. excessive administration of sodium bicarbonate (ref. pg. 268)
13. (ref. pg. 269)
    a. 7.23, 29
    b. 7.58, 17 or 18
    c. a combination of both
       a base deficit
       12–14 mEq/L
    d. respiratory
       a base excess
       3–4 mEq/L

CHAPTER EIGHT

VENTILATION-PERFUSION RELATIONSHIPS

VENTILATION-PERFUSION RATIO

1. 4 (ref. pg. 277)
2. 5 (ref. pg. 277)
3. 4 : 5, 0.8 (ref. pg. 277)
4. higher (ref. pg. 277)
5. lower (ref. pg. 278)
6. decreases (ref. pg. 278)
7. a. the amount of oxygen ventilated into the alveoli
   b. the amount of oxygen removal by capillary blood flow (ref. pg. 278)
8. a. the amount of carbon dioxide that diffuses into the alveoli from the capillary blood
   b. the amount of carbon dioxide removal out of the alveoli by means of ventilation (ref. pg. 278)
9. it washes out of the alveoli faster than it is replaced by the venous blood (ref. pg. 279)
10. it does not diffuse into the blood as fast as it enters the alveolus.
    The PA_{O_2} also increases because of the reduced PA_{CO_2} (ref. pg. 279)
11. a (ref. pg. 279)
12. oxygen moves out of the alveolus and into the pulmonary capillary blood faster than it is replenished by ventilation (ref. pg. 280)
13. it moves out of the capillary blood and into the alveolus faster than it is washed out of the alveolus (ref. pg. 280)
14. c (ref. pg. 280
15. decreases (ref. pg. 282)
16. increases (ref. pg. 282)
17. decreases (ref. pg. 283)
18. gas exchange between the systemic capillaries and the tissue cells (ref. pg. 284)
19. 250 (ref. pg. 284)
20. 200 (ref. pg. 284)
21. ratio between the volume of oxygen consumed and the volume of carbon dioxide produced (ref. pg. 284)
22. $RQ = \frac{\dot{V}_{CO_2}}{\dot{V}_{O_2}}$ (ref. pg. 285)

23. gas exchange between the pulmonary capillaries and the alveoli (ref. pg. 285)
24. quantity of oxygen and carbon dioxide exchanged during a period of 1 minute (ref. pg. 285)
25. a. pulmonary emboli
    b. partial or complete obstruction in the pulmonary artery or arterioles
    c. extrinsic pressure on the pulmonary vessels
    d. destruction of the pulmonary vessels
    e. decreased cardiac output (ref. pg. 285)
26. a. obstructive lung disorder
    b. restrictive lung disorders
    c. hypoventilation from any cause (ref. pg. 285)

CHAPTER NINE

CONTROL OF VENTILATION

THE RESPIRATORY COMPONENTS OF THE MEDULLA

1. a. dorsal respiratory group
   b. ventral respiratory group (ref. pg. 294)
2. a (ref. pg. 295)
3. c (ref. pg. 296)
4. b. (ref. pg. 296)
5. the lower pons (ref. pg. 296)
6. b (ref. pg. 297)
7. b (ref. pg. 297)

MONITORING SYSTEMS THAT INFLUENCE THE RESPIRATORY COMPONENTS OF THE MEDULLA

1. hydrogen ions $[H^+]$ (ref. pg. 298)
2. bilaterally and ventrally in the substance of the medulla (ref. pg. 298)
3. CO_2, H^+, HCO_3^- (ref. pg. 298)
4. $CO_2 + H_2O \rightleftarrows H_2CO_3 \rightleftarrows H^+ + HCO_3^-$ (ref. pg. 298)
5. The central chemoreceptors transmit signals to the respiratory component in the medulla, which, in turn, increases alveolar ventilation (ref. pg. 298)
6. indirect, pH level of the CSF (ref. pg. 299)
7. special oxygen-sensitive cells that react to reductions of oxygen levels in the arterial blood (ref. pg. 299)
8. high in the neck, at the bifurcation of the internal and external carotid arteries and on the aortic arch (ref. pg. 299)
9. glossopharyngeal (9th); vagus (10th) (ref. pg. 299)
10. a (ref. pg. 299)
11. 60 mm Hg (ref. pg. 300)
12. 30 mm Hg (ref. pg. 300)
13. A chronically high CO_2 concentration in the CSF inactivates the H^+ sensitivity of the central chemoreceptors. HCO_3^- moves into the CSF via the active transport mechanism and combines with H^+, thus returning the pH to normal. (ref. pg. 300)
14. a (ref. pg. 300)
15. a. chronic anemia
    b. carbon monoxide poisoning
    c. methemoglobinemia (ref. pg. 301)

16. a. decreased pH ($\uparrow H^+$ level)
    b. hypoperfusion
    c. increased temperature
    d. nicotine
    e. the direct effect of Pa_{CO_2} (ref. pg. 301)
17. a. peripheral vasoconstriction
    b. increased pulmonary vascular resistance
    c. systemic arterial hypertension
    d. tachycardia
    e. increase in left ventricular performance (ref. pg. 304)

REFLEXES THAT INFLUENCE VENTILATION

1. lung overinflation (ref. pg. 304)
2. inspiration to cease (ref. pg. 304)
3. lung compression or deflation (ref. pg. 304)
4. an increased rate of breathing (ref. pg. 304)
5. lung compression, or lung exposure to noxious gases (ref. pg. 304)
6. in the trachea, bronchi, and bronchioles (ref. pg. 304)
7. the ventilatory rate to increase (ref. pg. 304)
8. small conducting airways, blood vessels, and interstitial tissues between the pulmonary capillaries and alveolar walls (ref. pg. 305)
9. juxtapulmonary-capillary receptors, or J-receptors (ref. pg. 305)
10. alveolar inflammation, pulmonary capillary congestion and edema, humoral agents (e.g., serotonin and bradykinin), lung deflation, and emboli (ref. pg. 305)
11. rapid, shallow breathing pattern (ref. pg. 305)
12. muscles, tendons, joints, and pain receptors in muscles and skin (ref. pg. 305)
13. medulla; increased number of inspiratory signals (ref. pg. 305)
14. increased respiratory rate during exercise (ref. pg. 305)
15. greater (ref. pg. 305)
16. increase (ref. pg. 305)
17. increase (ref. pg. 305)
18. a decreased heart and ventilatory rate (ref. pg. 305)
19. an increased heart and ventilatory rate (ref. pg. 305)

CHAPTER TEN

FETAL DEVELOPMENT AND THE CARDIOPULMONARY SYSTEM

FETAL LUNG DEVELOPMENT

1. a. embryonic
   b. pseudoglandular
   c. canalicular
   d. terminal sac (ref. pg. 314)
2. 24th (ref. pg. 314)
3. 20 (ref. pg. 315)
4. 28th (ref. pg. 316)

PLACENTA

1. cotyledons (ref. pg. 316)
2. (Fig. 10-3, pg. 318)
3. umbilical arteries (ref. pg. 317)
4. 20, 55 (ref. pg. 317)
5. the decreased maternal P_{CO_2} is caused by the alveolar hyperventilation that develops as the growing infant restricts the mother's diaphragmatic excursion (ref. pg. 318)
6. a. maternal-fetal P_{O_2} gradient
   b. higher hemoglobin concentration in the fetal blood
   c. greater affinity of fetal hemoglobin for oxygen (ref. pg. 318)
7. 30, 40 (ref. pg. 319)
8. umbilical vein (ref. pg. 319)
9. a. the placenta itself is an actively metabolizing organ
   b. the permeability of the placenta varies from region to region with respect to respiratory gases
   c. the fetal and maternal vascular shunts (ref. pg. 319)

FETAL CIRCULATION

1. ductus venosus (ref. pg. 319)
2. foramen ovale (ref. pg. 319)
3. left ventricle, heart, brain (ref. pg. 319)
4. ductus arteriosus, aorta (ref. pg. 319)
5. 15, pulmonary veins (ref. pg. 319)
6. 20 (ref. pg. 319)

Matching

7. e
   c
   a
   b
   d (ref. pg. 319)
8. a. the placenta is passed by the mother
   b. the umbilical arteries atrophy and become the lateral umbilical ligaments
   c. the umbilical vein becomes the round ligament (ligamentum teres) of the liver
   d. the ductus venosus becomes the ligamentum venosum, which is a fibrous cord in the liver
   e. the flap on the foramen ovale usually closes and becomes a depression in the interatrial septum called the fossa ovalis
   f. the ductus arteriosus atrophies and becomes the ligamentum arteriosum (ref. pg. 319)
9. a. about one-third of the fluid is squeezed out of the lungs as the infant passes through the birth canal
   b. about one-third of the fluid is absorbed by the pulmonary capillaries
   c. about one-third of the fluid is removed by the lymphatic system (ref. pg. 321)
10. 24 (ref. pg. 321)
11. 12 (ref. pg. 321)

BIRTH

1. a. thermal
   b. tactile
   c. visual (ref. pg. 321)
2. −40 (ref. pg. 322)
3. 40 (ref. pg. 322)
4. 0.005 L/cm H_2O (ref. pg. 322)
5. 30 cm H_2O/L/sec (ref. pg. 322)
6. a. the sudden increase in the alveolar P_{O_2}, which offsets the hypoxic vasoconstriction
   b. the mechanical increase in lung volume, which widens the caliber of the extra-alveolar vessels (ref. pg. 323)
7. As the pulmonary vascular resistance decreases, a greater amount of blood flows through the lungs, and therefore more blood returns to the left atrium. This causes the pressure in the left atrium to increase and the flap of the foramen ovale to close. (ref. pg. 323)
8. 45, 50 (ref. pg. 323)

9. When the ductus arteriosus remains open (permitting blood to pass through it), and the pulmonary vascular resistance is elevated, persistent pulmonary hypertension of the neonate is said to exist (ref. pg. 323)
10. persistent fetal circulation (ref. pg. 323)
11. a. bradykinin
    b. serotonin
    c. prostaglandin inhibitors (ref. pg. 323)

CONTROL OF VENTILATION IN THE NEWBORN

1. peripheral, central (ref. pg. 323)
2. decrease (ref. pg. 324)
3. respiratory slowing or apnea (ref. pg. 324)
4. marked hyperventilation (ref. pg. 324)
5. a deep inspiration that is elicited by lung inflation (ref. pg. 324)

NORMAL CLINICAL PARAMETERS IN THE NEWBORN

1. (ref. pg. 325)
2. (ref. pg. 325)

CHAPTER ELEVEN

AGING AND THE CARDIOPULMONARY SYSTEM

THE INFLUENCE OF AGING ON THE RESPIRATORY SYSTEM

1. 20 (ref. pg. 335)
2. 20, 25 (ref. pg. 335)
3. decreases, increases (ref. pg. 336)
4. a. increases
   b. decreases
   c. decreases
   d. remains the same
   e. increases
   f. increases
   g. decreases (ref. pg. 338)
5. a. decreases
   b. decreases
   c. decreases
   d. decreases
   e. decreases
   f. decreases (ref. pg. 338)
6. a. decreases (ref. pg. 338)
   b. increases (ref. pg. 338)
   c. increases (ref. pg. 339)
   d. decreases (ref. pg. 339)
   e. remains the same (ref. pg. 339)
   f. remains the same (ref. pg. 339)
   g. remains the same (ref. pg. 339)
   h. decreases (ref. pg. 339)
   i. decreases (ref. pg. 339)

ARTERIAL BLOOD GASES

1. b (ref. pg. 339)
2. b (ref. pg. 339)

THE INFLUENCE OF AGING ON THE CARDIOVASCULAR SYSTEM

1. b (ref. pg. 340)
2. b (ref. pg. 341)
3. b (ref. pg. 341)
4. 150 (ref. pg. 342)
5. a. decreases (ref. pg. 342)
   b. decreases (ref. pg. 342)
   c. increases (ref. pg. 343)
   d. increases (ref. pg. 343)
   e. increases (ref. pg. 343)

CHAPTER TWELVE

ELECTROPHYSIOLOGY OF THE HEART

ELECTROPHYSIOLOGY OF THE HEART

1. action potentials (ref. pg. 349)
2. polarized or resting state (ref. pg. 349)
3. resting membrane potential (RMP) (ref. pg. 350)
4. potassium (K^+) sodium (Na^+), and calcium (Ca^{2+}). (ref. pg. 350)
5. greatest (ref. pg. 350)
6. K^+ cation; Na^+ cation (ref. pg. 350)
7. −90 mV (ref. pg. 351)
8. action potential (ref. pg. 351)

The Five Phases of the Action Potential

1. Na^+; Na^+ channels; positively charged (ref. pg. 351)
2. +30 mV; upstroke. (ref. pg. 351)
3. K^+; K^+; out (ref. pg. 351)
4. Downward (ref. pg. 351)
5. inward; Ca^{2+}; outward; K^+ (ref. pg. 351)
6. prolonged (ref. pg. 351)
7. inward; Ca^{2+}, outward; K^+ (ref. pg. 351)
8. Na^+ ; K^+; Na^+; K^+ (ref. pg. 351)

PROPERTIES OF THE CARDIAC MUSCLE

1. contractile muscle fibers; autorhythmic cells. (ref. pg. 352)
2. contractile fiber cells (ref. pg. 352)
3. sinoatrial node (ref. pg. 352)
4. into; 4 (ref. pg. 352)
5. more; less (ref. pg. 353)
6. transmit; cell to cell (ref. pg. 353)
7. shorten and contract (ref. pg. 353)

Refractory periods

1. cannot respond to a stimulus. (ref. pg. 353)
2. 0, 1, 2, and about half of phase 3 (ref. pg. 353)
3. strong (ref. pg. 353)
4. 3 (ref. pg. 354)
5. resting or polarized state (ref. pg. 354)
6. 4 (ref. pg. 354)

The Conductive System

1. See Figure 12-4, pg. 354

Autonomic Nervous System

1. heart rate, AV conduction, cardiac contractility, and excitability (ref. pg. 355)
2. heart rate, AV conduction, contractility, and excitability (ref. pg. 355)

CHAPTER THIRTEEN

THE STANDARD 12-ECG SYSTEM

THE STANDARD 12-ECG SYSTEM

1. four; six (ref. pg. 358)
2. See Table 13-1 in textbook (ref. pg. 358)
3. a. views the electrical activity of the heart from a different angle (ref. pg. 358)
   b. has a positive and negative component (ref. pg. 358)
   c. monitors specific portions of the heart from the point of view of the positive electrode in that lead (ref. pg. 358)

Standard Limb Leads

1. bipolar leads; positive; negative (ref. pg. 358)
2. axis (ref. pg. 358)
3. Einthoven's triangle (ref. pg. 358)
4. positive deflections (ref. pg. 358)
5. equiphasic; straight (ref. pg. 359)
6. Negative (ref. pg. 359)
7. base; apex; right; left (ref. pg. 359)
8. positive; zero; center; center; negative; electrode; center. (ref. pg. 361)
9. 50%; augmentation; voltage; positive electrode is placed (ref. pg. 361)
10. frontal plane; base to the apex of the heart; right; left (ref. pg. 361)
11. left lateral leads; inferior leads (ref. pg. 361)

Precordial (Chest) Leads

1. horizontal plane; right ventricle; ventricle septum; left ventricle (ref. pg. 361)
2. anterior leads; lateral leads (ref. pg. 362)

Modified Chest Lead

1. V1; left arm or left shoulder area (ref. pg. 364)

NORMAL ECG CONFIGURATIONS AND THEIR EXPECTED MEASUREMENTS (LEAD II)

The ECG Paper

1. 0.04; five; 0.20 (ref. pg. 364)
2. 5; 300 (ref. pg. 364)
3. amplitude; 0.1; 1 (ref. pg. 364)
4. 10 (ref. pg. 364)
5. 15; 3 (ref. pg. 364)
6. baseline; it changes into another wave form (ref. pg. 366)
7. Complex (ref. pg. 364)
8. Segment (ref. pg. 364)
9. Interval (ref. pg. 364)
10. positive; negative (ref. pg. 364)

The P wave

1. P-wave (ref. pg. 366)
2. symmetric; upright (ref. pg. 366)
3. AV node (ref. pg. 366)
4. flat; isoelectic (ref. pg. 366)
5. 0.08 to 0.11; 2–2 $^{1}/_{2}$ (ref. pg. 366)
6. 0.2 to 0.3; 2–3 (ref. pg. 366)
7. atrial abnormalities (ref. pg. 366)
8. ventricles are depolarizing (ref. pg. 366)

The P-R Interval

1. P-wave; QRS complex (ref. pg. 367)
2. 0.12 to 0.20; 3 to 5 (ref. pg. 367)
3. bundle of His, ventricular branches, and Purkinje fiber system (ref. pg. 367)

The QRS Complex

1. ventricular depolarization (ref. pg. 367)
2. Q wave, R wave, and S wave (ref. pg. 367)
3. Q wave (ref. pg. 367)
4. R wave (ref. pg. 367)
5. S (ref. pg. 367)
6. 0.10; 2 $^{1}/_{2}$ (ref. pg. 367)
7. longer; 0.10 (ref. pg. 367)
8. premature ventricular contractions (PVCs), increased amplitude, and T waves of opposite polarity (ref. pg. 367)

The ST Segment

1. ventricular depolarization and repolarization (ref. pg. 368)
2. QRS complex (called the J point); T wave (ref. pg. 368)
3. 0.12 (ref. pg. 368)
4. Ischemia (ref. pg. 368)

The T Wave

1. ventricular repolarization, rest, and recovery (ref. pg. 369)
2. 0.5 (ref. pg. 369)
3. 0.20 (ref. pg. 369)
4. refractory period (ref. pg. 369)
5. relative refractory (ref. pg. 369)
6. acid-base imbalances, hyperventilation, hyperkalemia, and the presence of various drugs (ref. pg. 369)

The U Wave

1. T wave; T wave (ref. pg. 369)
2. flat and not seen (ref. pg. 369)

The QT Interval

1. QRS complex; T wave (ref. pg. 370)
2. total ventricular activity — that is, ventricular depolarization (QRS) and repolarization (ST segment and the T wave (ref. pg. 370)
3. 0.38 (ref. pg. 370)
4. 40 (ref. pg. 370)
5. indirectly (ref. pg. 370)

CHAPTER FOURTEEN

ECG INTERPRETATION

STEP ONE: DOES THE GENERAL APPEARANCE OF THE ECG TRACING APPEAR NORMAL OR ABNORMAL?

1. Closely scan the ECG tracing and identify each of the wave components. Note any specific wave abnormalities. Are there any abnormalities—in terms of appearance or duration—in the P-waves, QRS complexes, ST segments, or T waves? Do the complexes appear consistent from one beat to the next? Does the rate appear too slow or too fast? Does the rhythm appear regular or irregular? Are there any extra beats or pauses? It is often helpful to circle any possible abnormalities during step one. This initial process helps to pinpoints problems areas that can be inspected more carefully during the steps discussed below. (ref. pg. 374)

STEP TWO: DOES THE VENTRICULAR ACTIVITY (QRS COMPLEXES) APPEAR NORMAL OR ABNORMAL?

Rate

1. large; QRS complexes; 300; large (ref. pg. 375)
2. See Table 14-1 (ref. pg. 374)
3. vertical 3-second marks (ref. pg. 375)
4. 6-second interval (two 3-second marks); 10 (ref. pg. 375)

Rhythm

1. shortest; longest (ref. pg. 375)
2. 0.12 (ref. pg. 375)

Shape

1. 0.10; 2 1/2 small squares or less (ref. pg. 376)
2. supraventricular origin (ref. pg. 376)
3. 0.10; distorted (ref. pg. 376)

STEP THREE: DOES THE ATRIAL ACTIVITY APPEAR NORMAL OR ABNORMAL?

1. QRS complexes (ref. pg. 376)
2. the same (ref. pg. 376)
3. QRS rhythm; P-P intervals (ref. pg. 376)
4. P-waves that are not of expected polarity, atrial flutter, fibrillation, or P prime (P′) waves (i.e., waves initiated by the atrial, not the SA node) (ref. pg. 376)

STEP FOUR: DOES THE ATRIOVENTRICULAR RELATIONSHIP APPEAR NORMAL?

1. all the atrial impulses (ref. pg. 376)
2. a. Is each P-wave followed by a QRS complex? (ref. pg. 377)
   b. Is each QRS complex preceded by a single P-wave? (ref. pg. 377)
3. 0.20 (ref. pg. 377)

STEP FIVE: WHAT IS THE ECG INTERPRETATION?

1. (ref. pg. 377)

P-wave	The P-waves are positive (upright) and uniform. A QRS complex follows every P-wave.
P-R Interval:	The duration of the P-R interval is between 0.12 and 0.20 second and is constant from beat to beat.
QRS Complex	The duration of the QRS complex is 0.10 second or less. A P-wave precedes every QRS complex.
QRS Rate:	Between 60 and 100 beats per minute.
QRS Rhythm:	Regular

THE SINUS MECHANISMS

Sinus Bradycardia

1. slow (ref. pg. 378)
2. 60 (ref. pg. 378)
3. (ref. pg. 378)

P-wave:	The P-waves are positive and uniform. Each P-wave is followed by a QRS complex.
P-R Interval:	The P-R interval has a normal duration between 0.12 and 0.20 second and is constant from beat to beat.

QRS Complex: The QRS complex duration is 0.10 second or less. A P-wave precedes every QRS complex.
QRS Rate: Less than 60 beats per minute.
QRS Rhythm: Regular

4. a weakened or damaged sinoatrial (SA) node, severe or chronic hypoxemia, increased intracranial pressure, obstructive sleep apnea, and certain drugs (most notably the beat-blockers) (ref. pg. 379)
5. decreased; lowered (ref. pg. 379)
6. decreased; hypoxia (ref. pg. 379)

Sinus Tachycardia

1. fast (ref. pg. 379)
2. 100, 160 (ref. pg. 379)
3. (ref. pg. 379)

   P-wave: The P-waves are positive and uniform. Each P-wave is followed by a QRS complex.
   P-R interval: The P-R interval has a normal duration between 0.12 and 0.20 second and is constant from beat to beat.
   QRS complex: The QRS complex duration is 0.10 second or less. A P-wave precedes every QRS compex.
   QRS Rate: Between 100 and 160 beats per minute.
   QRS Rhythm: Regular
4. exercise, emotions, fever, pain, fear, anger, and anxiety (ref. pg. 380)
5. hypoxemia, hypovolemia, severe anemia, hyperthermia, massive hemorrhage, hyperthyroidism, and any condition that leads to an increased sympathetic stimulation (ref. pg. 380)
6. congestive heart failure, cardiogenic shock, myocardial ischemia, heart valve disorders, pulmonary embolism, hypertension, and infarction (ref. pg. 380)

Sinus Arrhythmia

1. 10 (ref. pg. 380)
2. normal (ref. pg. 380)
3. (ref. pg. 380)

   P-wave: The P-waves are positive and uniform. Each P-wave is followed by a QRS complex.
   P-R Interval: The P-R interval has a normal duration between 0.12 and 0.20 second and is constant from beat to beat.
   QRS Complex: The QRS complex duration is 0.10 second or less. A P-wave precedes every QRS complex.
   QRS Rate: Varies by more than 10 percent. It is helpful to report the rate range.
   QRS Rhythm: Irregular
4. children; young adults. (ref. pg. 380)

Sinus (SA) Block

1. sinus exit block; blocked. (ref. pg. 381)
2. at the precise time it would normally appear if the sinus block had not occurred (ref. pg. 381)
3. (ref. pg. 381)

P-wave:	The P-waves are positive and uniform. However, there is an entire P-QRS-T complex missing.
P-R Interval:	The P-R interval has a normal duration between 0.12 and 0.20 second and is constant from beat to beat, except for the pause when an entire cycle is missing. The P-R interval may be slightly shorter after the pause.
QRS Complex:	Except for the missing cycle, the QRS complex duration is 0.10 second or less, and a P-wave precedes every QRS complex.
QRS Rate:	The rate may vary according to the number and position of missing P-QRS-T cycles.
QRS Rhythm:	The rhythm may be regular or irregular according to the number and position of missing P-QRS-T cycles.

Sinus Arrest

1. sudden failure of the SA node to initiate an impulse (i.e., no P-wave) (ref. pg. 382)
2. (ref. pg. 382)

P-wave:	No P-wave.
P-R Interval:	The P-R interval has a normal duration between 0.12 and 0.20 second and is constant from beat to beat.
QRS complex:	The QRS complex duration is 0.10 second or less. After a sinus arrest, however, the QRS duration may be greater than 0.10 second when the escape rhythm is initiated by the AV node.
QRS Rate:	Normal sinus rhythm during non-sinus arrest periods.
QRS Rhythm:	The QRS complexes before and after the sinus arrest are regular. The escape rate may be regular or irregular.

THE ATRIAL MECHANISMS

Premature Atrial Complex (PAC)

1. abnormal electrical activity in the atria cause the atria to depolarize before the SA node fires (ref. pg. 382)
2. ectopic foci (ref. pg. 382)
3. prime (P′) (ref. pg. 382)
4. (ref. pg. 383)

P-wave:	The P′-wave will appear different from a normal SA node induced P-save. When the PAC is early, the P′ may be hidden, or partially hidden, in the preceding T wave. P′-waves hidden in the T wave often distort, or increase the

	amplitude of the T wave. A PAC may not successfully into the ventricles if the AV node or bundle branches are in their complete refractory period. This is called a *blocked* or *nonconducted* PAC.
P-R Interval:	The P′-R interval may be normal or prolonged, depending on the timing of the PAC. Most often, however, the P′-R interval is different from the normal SA node rhythm.
QRS Complex:	Except for the cycle that is missing, the QRS complex duration is 0.10 second or less, and a P-wave precedes every QRS complex.
QRS Rate:	Varies
QRS Rhythm:	Irregular

5. impending heart failure, right coronary artery disease, digitalis excess, pericarditis, ingestion of stimulants, caffeine, and recreational drug abuse (ref. pg. 383)
6. a. patients with chronic pulmonary lung disease (ref. pg. 383)
   b. females during the third trimester of pregnancy (ref. pg. 383)

Atrial Bigeminy

1. every other beat is an ectopic atrial beat—a PAC (ref. pg. 383)
2. congestive heart failure. (ref. pg. 384)

Atrial Tachycardia

1. 130 to 250 (ref. pg. 384)
2. paroxysmal atrial tachycardia (ref. pg. 384)
3. (ref. pg. 385)

P-wave:	Starts abruptly, at rates of 130 to 250 beats per minute. The P′-wave may or may not be seen. Visible P′-saves differ in configuration from the normal sinus P-wave. At more rapid rates, the P′ is hidden in the preceding T wave and cannot be seen as a separate entity.
P-R Interval:	The P-R interval has a normal duration between 0.12 and 0.20 second and is constant from beat to beat. The P′-R interval is difficult to measure at rapid rates.
QRS Complex:	The QRS complex duration is 0.10 second or less. A P-wave usually precedes every QRS complex, although a 2:1 AV conduction ratio is often seen. The QRS complexes during atrial tachycardia may be normal or abnormal, depending on the degree of ventricular refractoriness and AV conduction time.
QRS Rate:	Very regular
QRS Rhythm:	Atrial trachycardia begins suddenly and is very regular.

4. anxiety, caffeine, smoking, and excessive alcohol ingestion (ref. pg. 385)

Atrial Flutter

1. two or more regular "sawtooth-like" waves, called *flutter* or *ff waves* (ref. pg. 385)
2. 200, 300 (ref. pg. 385)

3. (ref. pg. 386)

ff Waves:	Atrial depolarization is regular. Commonly has a "sawtooth" or "sharktooth" like appearance.
P-R Interval:	The P′-R interval of the *ff* waves is typically between 0.24 to 0.40 second and consistent with the QRS complex.
QRS Complex:	The QRS complex duration is usually 0.10 second or less. Depending on the degree of ventricular refractoriness, the QRS may be greater than 0.10 second. When this is the case, the ff waves distort the QRS complexes and T waves.
QRS Rate:	The QRS rate is a function of the degree of ventricular refractoriness and of the AV conduction time.
QRS Rhythm:	Depending on AV conduction, the QRS rhythm may be regular or irregular.

4. 40 years of age, chronic obstructive pulmonary disease (e.g., emphysema or chronic bronchitis), chronic heart disease (e.g., congestive heart failure or valvular heart disease), chronic hypertension, myocardial ischemia, myocardial infarction, hyoxemia, quinidine excess, pulmonary embolus, and hepatic disease (ref. pg. 386)

Atrial Fibrillation

1. disorganized and ineffective state within the atria (ref. pg. 386)
2. coarse fibrillation (ref. pg. 386)
3. 300, 600 (ref. pg. 387)
4. *fib* or *ff* waves. (ref. pg. 387)
5. (ref. pg. 388)

ff Waves:	Atrial depolarization is chaotic and irregular
P-R Interval:	There are no P-R intervals.
QRS Complex:	The QRS complex duration is usually 0.10 second or less. The *ff* waves often distort the QRS complexes and T waves.
QRS Rate:	The QRS rate is a function of the degree of ventricular refractoriness and conduction time.
QRS Rhythm:	Depending on AV conduction, the QRS rhythm may be regular or irregular.

6. chronic pulmonary disease, valvular heart disease, congestive heart failure, ischemic heart disease, and hypertensive heart disorders (ref. pg. 388)
7. emotional stress, excessive alcohol consumption, and excessive straining and vomiting (ref. pg. 388)

THE VENTRICULAR MECHANISMS

Premature Ventricular Complex (PVC)

1. abnormal electrical activity arising within the ventricles (ref. pg. 388)
2. (ref. pg. 388)

P-wave:	There is no P-wave before a PVC. The P-waves of the dominant rhythm are normal.
P-R Interval:	There is no P-R interval before a PVC. The P-R intervals of the dominant rhythm are normal.

QRS Complex:	The QRS complex is wide (long duration), bizarre, and unlike the normal QRS complex. The QRS of the PVC usually has an increased amplitude with a T wave of opposite polarity. The QRS/T may also present with diminished amplitude and narrow duration.
QRS Rate:	The QRS rate is that of the underlying rhythm
QRS Rhythm:	The rhythm is that of the underlying rhythm, and PVCs disturb the regularity.

3. uniform PVCs; multiform PVCs, paried PVCs, bigeminal PVCs, and trigeminal PVCs. (ref. pg. 389)
4. from one focus; appearance, size and amplitude (ref. pg. 389)
5. more than one focus; shapes and amplitudes (ref. pg. 389)
6. two closely coupled PVCs in a row (ref. pg. 389)
7. every other beat—that is, a normal sinus beat, PVC, sinus beat, PVC, and so on (ref. pg. 389)
8. when every third beat is a PVC (ref. pg. 389)
9. intrinsic myocardial disease, electrolyte disturbances, hypoxemia, acidemia, hypokalemia, hypertension, hypovolemia, stress, and congestive heart failure (ref. pg. 389)
10. digitalis, isoproterenol, dopamine, epinephrine, and caffeine. PVCs may also be a sign of theophylline or alpha-or beta-agonist toxicity. (ref. pg. 389)

Ventricular Tachycardia

1. ventricular tachycardia (ref. pg. 389)
2. 100, 170 (ref. pg. 389)
3. paroxysmal or intermittent (ref. pg. 391)
4. sustained ventricular tachycardia or V-tach (ref. pg. 391)
5. decreased (ref. pg. 391)
6. (ref. pg. 391)

P-wave	The P-wave usually cannot be identified during ventricular tachycardia.
P-R Interval:	The P-R interval cannot be measured.
QRS Complex:	The QRS duration is usually greater than 0.12 second and bizarre in appearance. The T wave usually cannot be identified.
QRS Rate:	Between 100 and 170 beats per minute. Three or more consecutive PVCs constitute ventricular tachycardia.
QRS Rhythm:	Regular or slightly irregular.

Ventricular Flutter

1. wide sine wave (regular, smooth, rounded ventricular wave) (ref. pg. 392)
2. 250, 350 (ref. pg. 392)
3. (ref. pg. 392)

P-wave:	The P-wave is usually not distinguishable.
P-R Interval:	The P-R interval is not measurable.
QRS Complex:	The QRS duration is usually greater than 0.12 second and bizarre in appearance. The T wave is usually not separated from the QRS complex.
QRS Rate:	Between 250 and 350 beats per minute
QRS Rhythm:	Regular or slightly irregular.

Ventricular Fibrillation

1. multiple and chaotic electrical activities of the ventricles (ref. pg. 392)
2. terminal (ref. pg. 392)
3. (ref. pg. 392)

P-wave:	The P-waves cannot be identified.
P-R Interval:	The P-R interval is not measurable.
QRS Complex:	The QRS complex cannot be identified.
QRS Rate:	A rate cannot be calculated.
QRS Rhythm:	The rhythm is chaotic because of multiple, disorganized ventricular contractions.

Asystole (Cardiac Standstill)

1. complete absence of electrical and mechanical activity (ref. pg. 393)
2. a flat line; severe damage to the heart's electrical conduction system (ref. pg. 393)

AV CONDUCTION DEFECTS

Sinus Rhythm with First-degree AV Block

1. increases (ref. pg. 394)
2. first-degree AV block (ref. pg. 394)
3. (ref. pg. 394)

P-wave:	The P-waves are positive and uniform. Each P-wave is followed by a QRS complex.
P-R Interval:	The P-R interval is consistently greater than 0.20 second from beat to beat.
QRS Complex:	The duration of the QRS complex is 0.10 second or less. Each QRS complex is preceded by a P-wave.
QRS Rate:	The rate is usually based upon the normal sinus rhythm and is constant between 60 and 100 per minute.
QRS Rhythm:	The rhythm is dependent on the sinus rhythm. When a sinus arrhythmia is present, the rhythm will vary accordingly.

4. right coronary artery disease, endocarditis, myocarditis, electrolyte disturbances, and advancing age (ref. pg. 395)

Sinus Rhythm with Second-degree AV Block, The Wenckebach Phenomenon

1. progressive delay in the conduction of the atrial impulse through the AV node until, eventually, an atrial impulse is completely blocked from the ventricles (ref. pg. 395)
2. Progressive prolongation of the P-R interval (ref. pg. 395)
   The complex Wenckebach cycle begins and ends with a P-wave
   There is one more P-wave than QRS complexes in a cycle

The appearance of all the P-R intervals after the missed QRS complex are the same, regardless of the numbers of P-QRS-T complexes in the cycle
Irregular or decreasing R-R intervals

Sinus Rhythm with Complete AV Block

1. blocked (ref. pg. 396)
2. His bundle; 40 to 60, junctional escape pacemaker. (ref. pg. 396)
3. Ventricular escape mechanism (ref. pg. 396)
4. 20 and 40 (ref. pg. 396)
5. (ref. pg. 396)

P-wave:	The P-waves are positive and uniform. There is no relationship between the P-waves and the QRS complexes. The atrial rate is faster than the ventricular escape rate.
P-R interval:	There is no measurable P-R intervals, as there is no relationship between the P-waves and QRS complexes.
QRS Complex:	The duration of the QRS complex may be normal, or greater than 0.12 second. When the pathology is above the His bundle, the QRS complex is usually normal (0.10 or less). When the pathology is below the His bundle, the duration of the QRS complexes will be greater than 0.12 second.
QRS Rate:	The atrial rate is faster and completely independent of the ventricular rate. A junctional escape pacemaker produces a rate between 40 and 60 beats per minute. A ventricular escape pacemaker produces a rate between 20 and 40 beats per minute.
QRS Rhythm:	Both a junctional escape pacemaker or a ventricular escape pacemaker produce a regular rhythm.

CHAPTER FIFTEEN

HEMODYNAMIC MONITORING

HEMODYNAMIC MEASUREMENTS DIRECTLY OBTAINED BY MEANS OF THE PULMONARY ARTERY CATHETER

1. the study of the forces that influence the circulation of blood (ref. pg. 403)
2. (ref. pg. 405)

HEMODYNAMIC VALUES COMPUTED FROM DIRECT MEASUREMENTS

1. (ref. pg. 405)
2. the volume of blood ejected by the ventricles with each contraction (ref. pg. 405)
3. a. preload
   b. afterload
   c. myocardial contractility (ref. pg. 405)
4. $SV = \frac{CO}{HR}$ (ref. pg. 406)
5. 63.21 ml/beat (ref. pg. 406)
6. dividing the stroke volume (SV) by the body surface area (BSA) (ref. pg. 407)
7. 22 ml/beat/m^2 (ref. pg. 407)
8. a. contractility of the heart
   b. overall blood volume status
   c. degree of venous return (ref. pg. 407)
9. dividing the cardiac output (CO) by the body's surface area (BSA) (ref. pg. 407)
10. 2.8 L/min/m^2 (ref. pg. 407)
11. the amount of work required by the right ventricle to pump blood (ref. pg. 407)
12. contractility of the right ventricle (ref. pg. 407)
13. $RVSWI = SVI \times (\overline{PA} - CVP) \times 0.0136$ g/ml (ref. pg. 408)
14. 8.16 g mm (ref. pg. 408)
15. the amount of work required by the left ventricle to pump blood (ref. pg. 408)
16. contractility of the left ventricle (ref. pg. 408)
17. $LVSWI = SVI \times (MAP - PCWP) \times 0.0136$ g/ml (ref. pg. 408)
18. 70.38 g m/m^2 (ref. pg. 408)
19. (ref. pg. 406)
20. low (ref. pg. 409)

21. high (ref. pg. 409)
22. the afterload of the right ventricle (ref. pg. 409)
23. $PVR = \frac{\overline{PA} - PCWP \times 80}{CO}$ (ref. pg. 409)
24. 114 dynes × sec cm^{-5} (ref. pg. 409)
25. (ref. pg. 410)
26. (ref. pg. 411)
27. the afterload of the left ventricle (ref. pg. 409)
28. $SVR = \frac{MAP - CVP \times 80}{CO}$ (ref. pg. 409)
29. 1266 dynes × sec cm^{-5} (ref. pg. 409)
30. (ref. pg. 411)

CHAPTER SIXTEEN

RENAL FAILURE AND ITS EFFECTS ON THE CARDIOPULMONARY SYSTEM

THE KIDNEYS

1. (ref. Fig. 16-2, pg. 420)
2. (ref. Fig. 16-3, pg. 422)
3. (ref. Fig. 16-4, pg. 423)

URINE FORMATION

1. (ref. pgs. 421–424)
2. a. proximal convoluted tubule
   b. loop of Henle
   c. distal convoluted tubule (ref. pg. 424)
3. proximal convoluted tubule (ref. pg. 424)
4. various substances are transported from the plasma of the peritubular capillaries to the fluid of the renal tubule (ref. pg. 424)
5. hydrogen (H^+), potassium (K^+) (ref. pg. 424)

URINE CONCENTRATION AND VOLUME

1. a. countercurrent mechanism
   b. selective permeability of the collecting duct (ref. pg. 425)
2. renal medulla (ref. pg. 425)
3. 300 (ref. pg. 425)
4. 300, 1200 (ref. pg. 425)
5. hypothalamus, pituitary gland (ref. pg. 425)
6. b (ref. pg. 425)
7. a (ref. pg. 425)
8. increases (ref. pg. 425)
9. decreases (ref. pg. 425)
10. 1.018 to 1.040 (ref. pg. 425)

REGULATION OF ELECTROLYTE CONCENTRATION

1. a. sodium
   b. potassium
   c. calcium, magnesium, and phosphate (ref. pg. 426)
2. hydrogen (ref. pg. 428)
3. sodium bicarbonate (ref. pg. 428)
4. a. capillary fluid shift system
   b. the renal system (ref. pg. 428)

RENAL FAILURE

1. a. unilateral renal agenesis
   b. renal dysplasia
   c. polycystic disease of the kidney (ref. pg. 429)
2. women (ref. pg. 429)
3. a. calculi
   b. normal pregnancy
   c. prostatic hypertrophy
   d. infection and inflammation causing scar tissue
   e. neurologic disorders (ref. Table 16-2, pg. 430)
4. a. altered immune responses
   b. drugs and related chemicals
   c radiation (ref. pg. 430)
5. Wilms' tumor (ref. pg. 430)
6. a. hypovolemia
   b. septicemia
   c. heart failure
   d. renal artery atherosclerosis (ref. Table 16-3, pg. 431)
7. a sharp reduction in urine output (ref. pg. 431)
8. a renal ischemia
   b. injury to the glomerular membrane caused by nephrotoxic agents
   c. acute tubular necrosis
   d. intratubular obstruction
   e. acute inflammatory conditions (ref. Table 16-4, pg. 431
9. a. ureteral obstruction (ref. Table 16-5, pg. 432)
   b. bladder outlet obstruction
10. decreases (ref. pg. 432)
11. increases (ref. pg. 432)
12. a (ref. pg. 432)
13. b (ref. pg. 432)

CARDIOPULMONARY PROBLEMS CAUSED BY RENAL FAILURE

1. sodium (ref. pg. 432)
2. a. increases
   b. increases
   c. decreases (ref. pg. 433)
3. b (ref. pg. 433)
4. b (ref. pg. 433)
5. a (ref. pg. 433)
6. a (ref. pg. 433)
7. a. the production of erythropoietin is often inadequate to stimulate the production of red blood cells
   b. toxic waste accumulation suppresses the ability of bone marrow to produce red blood cells (ref. pg. 433)
8. because of the platelet abnormalities associated with renal failure (ref. pg. 433)
9. this condition develops as a result of the exposure of the pericardium to the metabolic end-products associated with renal decline (ref. pg. 434)

CHAPTER SEVENTEEN

EXERCISE AND ITS EFFECTS ON THE CARDIOPULMONARY SYSTEM

EFFECTS OF EXERCISE

1. a. 20
   b. 3
   c. 6
   d. 25
   e. 20
   f. 20 (ref. pg. 443)
2. 30, 60 (ref. pg. 443)
3. 30, 50 (ref. pg. 443)
4. 40 (ref. pg. 444)
5. anaerobic threshold (ref. pg. 444)

VENTILATION

1. a. The cerebral cortex sending neural signals to the exercising muscles may also send collateral signals to the medulla oblongata to increase the rate and depth of breathing.
   b. Proprioceptors in the moving muscles, tendons, and joints transmitting sensory signals via the spinal cord to the respiratory centers of the medulla.
   c. The increase in body temperature during exercise contributing to increased ventilation. (ref. pg. 444)
2. e (ref. pg. 444)
3. depth, rate (ref. pg. 444)
4. depth, frequency (rate) (ref. pg. 444)
5. e (ref. pg. 444)
6. a. an increase in alveolar ventilation, within seconds after the onset of exercise.
   b. a slow, gradual further increase in alveolar ventilation developing over approximately the first 3 minutes of exercise.
   c. alveolar ventilation stabilizes. (ref. pgs. 444, 445)
7. 50, 65 (ref. pg. 445)
8. 250 (ref. pg. 446)
9. 95 (ref. pg. 446)

10. c (ref. pg. 446)
11. increased cardiac output (ref. pg. 447)
12. d (ref. pgs. 447, 448)

CIRCULATION

1. a. sympathetic discharge
   b. increase in cardiac output
   c. increase in arterial blood pressure (ref. pgs. 448, 449)
2. a. The heart is stimulated to increase its rate and strength of contraction
   b. The blood vessels of the peripheral vascular system constrict, except for the blood vessels of the working muscles, which dilate (ref. pg. 449)
3. an increased cardiac output (ref. pg. 450)
4. a. an increased stroke volume
   b. an increased heart rate
   c. combination of both (ref. pg. 450)
5. vasodilation (ref. pg. 450)
6. Frank-Starling (ref. pg. 451)
7. 165 (ref. pg. 451)
8. increases, decreases (ref. pg. 452)
9. a. the individual's physical condition
   b. the specific muscles that are working
   c. the distribution of blood flow (ref. pg. 452)
10. decreases (ref. pg. 452)
11. a. the sympathetic discharge
    b. the increased cardiac output
    c. the vasoconstriction of the blood vessels in the non-working muscle areas. (ref. pg. 452)
12. a. increases
    b. increases
    c. increases
    d. increases (ref. pg. 452)
13. local vasodilators (ref. pg. 452)

STROKE VOLUME VERSUS HEART RATE IN INCREASING THE CARDIAC OUTPUT

1. heart rate, increased stroke volume (ref. pg. 455)
2. 50 (ref. pg. 455)
3. increased heart rate (ref. pg. 455)
4. 65 (ref. pg. 455)

BODY TEMPERATURE/CUTANEOUS BLOOD FLOW RELATIONSHIP

1. profuse sweating, followed by no sweating; extreme weakness; muscle cramping; exhaustion; nausea; headache; dizziness; confusion; staggering gait; unconsciousness; circulatory collapse (ref. pg. 456)
2. a. Spraying cool water on the victim's body
   b. Continually sponging the victim with cool water
   c. Blowing air over the body with a strong fan
   d. A combination of all three (ref. pgs. 456, 457)

CARDIOVASCULAR REHABILITATION

1. a. acute, in-hospital
   b. outpatient, immediately after hospitalization
   c. long-term outpatient
   d. maintenance (ref. pg. 457)

CHAPTER EIGHTEEN

HIGH ALTITUDE AND ITS EFFECTS ON THE CARDIOPULMONARY SYSTEM

EFFECTS OF HIGH ALTITUDE

1. 18,000–19,000 (ref. pg. 461)
2. increased alveolar ventilation (ref. pg. 463)
3. six weeks (ref. pg. 463)
4. c (ref. pg. 464)
5. c (ref. pg. 464)
6. 20–25% greater (ref. pg. 464)
7. a (ref. pg. 464)
8. increased (ref. pg. 464)
9. c (ref. pgs. 464, 465)
10. a (ref. pg. 465)

OTHER PHYSIOLOGIC CHANGES

1. a (ref. pg. 467)
2. headache, fatigue, dizziness, palpitation, nausea, loss of appetite, and insomnia (ref. pg. 467)
3. second or third day after ascent (ref. pgs. 467, 468)
4. vasoconstriction; increased (ref. pg. 468)
5. photophobia, ataxia, hallucinations, clouding of consciousness, coma, and possibly death (ref. pg. 468)
6. fatigue, reduced exercise tolerance, headache, dizziness, somnolence, loss of mental acuity, marked polycythemia, and severe hypoxemia (ref. pg. 468)

CHAPTER NINETEEN

HIGH-PRESSURE ENVIRONMENTS AND THEIR EFFECTS ON THE CARDIOPULMONARY SYSTEM

DIVING

1. 1.0 atmosphere (ref. pg. 471)
2. a. 1.375 liters (ref. pgs. 471, 472)
   b. 3040 mm Hg (ref. Figure 19-1, pg. 473)
3. a. the diver's metabolic rate
   b. the diver's ability to store and transport O_2 and CO_2 (ref. pg. 472)
4. 55 (ref. pg. 472)
5. descends, ascends (ref. pg. 474)
6. hypoxia of ascent (ref. pg. 474)
7. a. bradycardia
   b. decreased cardiac output
   c. peripheral vasoconstriction (ref. pg. 474)
8. a. joint pains (the bends)
   b. chest pain and coughing (the chokes)
   c. paresthesia and paralysis (spinal cord involvement)
   d. circulatory failure
   e. death (severe cases) (ref. pg. 475)

HYPERBARIC MEDICINE

1. (ref. Table 19-1, pg. 477)
2. a. increases the physically dissolved O_2 in the arterial blood
   b. increases the pressure gradient for driving oxygen into ischemic tissues
   c. reduces the half-life of carboxyhemoglobin (CO_{Hb}) (ref. pg. 476)
3. 1 hour (ref. pg. 476)